LOWERING CHOLESTEROL IS EASY!!!
DID YOU KNOW?

* It's not butter . . . it's better! Discover the astonishing heart benefits of olive oil and the new stanol-containing margarine.

*You don't have to run a marathon . . . just a little gentle exercise every day can *substantially* improve your cholesterol profile.

*You don't have to eat tofu . . . these days you can choose from dozens of soy-based products to send your cholesterol south.

*You don't have to act like a nut . . . eat them instead. Both almonds and walnuts contain heart-healthy fats that can keep your arteries clear. So indulge!

*You can "pop a pill" . . . taking just a few nutritional supplements can make your "bad" cholesterol levels plummet—and energize you, too.

*You can break away from fast food. With *Outsmart High Cholesterol*, you can switch to healthier, more satisfying fare. It's simpler than you think, and it will take off unwanted pounds, too!

OUTSMART HIGH CHOLESTEROL

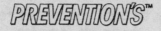

Outsmart
High Cholesterol

Also by the Editors of *Prevention* Health Books

The Ice Cream Diet

The Peanut Butter Diet

Anti-Aging Secrets

Complementary Cures

Energy Boosters

Pain-Free Living for Seniors

Fat Fighters

Healing Herbs

Natural Remedies for Women

Power Foods

Vitamin Cures

Available from St. Martin's Paperbacks

PREVENTION'S™

Outsmart High Cholesterol

EXPERT-ENDORSED STRATEGIES FOR HEART-HEALTHY CHOLESTEROL LEVELS—WITHOUT PRESCRIPTION DRUGS!

The Editors of *Prevention* Health Books

St. Martin's Paperbacks

ISBN: 0-312-98810-9
EAN: 80312-98810-4

Printed in the United States of America

Rodale / St. Martin's Paperbacks edition / March 2003

St. Martin's Paperbacks are published by St. Martin's Press, 175 Fifth Avenue, New York, NY 10010.

15 14 13 12 11 10 9 8 7

Visit us on the web at www.prevention.com

NOTICE

This book is intended as a reference volume only, not as a medical manual. The information given here is designed to help you make informed decisions about your health. It is not intended as a substitute for any treatment or dietary advice that may have been prescribed by your doctor. If you suspect that you have a medical problem, we urge you to seek competent medical care. If you have not participated in an exercise program regularly or recently, we encourage you to work with your physician to determine the activity level that is best for you.

Mention of specific companies, organizations, or authorities in this book does not imply endorsement by the publisher, nor does mention of specific companies, organizations, or authorities imply that they endorse the book.

Any Internet addresses and telephone numbers were accurate at the time the book went to press.

CONTENTS

INTRODUCTION

INTRODUCTION

Make no mistake: Even though you can't feel it or see it, high cholesterol is a serious problem. It can silently do its dirty work inside your arteries, building up plaques that can eventually block bloodflow to your heart or brain and trigger a heart attack or stroke.

If you have high cholesterol or these other conditions it can cause, you're certainly not alone. According to the American Heart Association, high cholesterol affects more than 100 million Americans. Many of them probably don't know it because they're not getting their cholesterol checked as often as they should. And those who have been diagnosed may not be managing their cholesterol effectively because they're not sure how to keep it under control.

Heart disease is the leading cause of death in the United States. In fact, if you're a woman, you're almost twice as likely to die of heart disease as cancer. And stroke takes the number three position in the leading causes of death in America.

Is this scary? Yes. But is it unavoidable? No.

You can start protecting yourself from becoming a statistic right now by taking your first step on a straightforward journey that leads to lower cholesterol and a healthier life.

This book contains the latest information from top heart experts on how to make your cholesterol plunge by making smart eating choices, losing weight, and getting adequate exercise. Sound difficult? It's not once you know how to do it right. In these pages, you'll find delicious recipes to use in the kitchen, advice for dropping those pounds once and for all, and suggestions on how to make exercise an enjoyable part of your life.

You'll also learn the best way to use vitamins, minerals, and other supplements in your fight against cholesterol. And you'll meet a number of people just like you who made these kinds of improvements and no longer live with the threat of unhealthy cholesterol.

Deciding to make these changes is a smart choice indeed. And with the information you're about to learn, your high cholesterol shouldn't stand a chance.

PART I

You *Can* Outsmart Cholesterol

CHAPTER ONE

Why Cholesterol Matters

Once upon a time, when red meat, whole milk, and creamery butter were favored fare in our country, high cholesterol got about as much attention from doctors and their patients as crow's-feet. It was interesting, but nothing to be alarmed about.

Not anymore. Doctors now know that high cholesterol can set the stage for a host of potentially debilitating health problems, including heart attack and stroke.

To add insult to injury, high cholesterol has a nasty way of sneaking up on you. If you've been ambushed by a sneak attack, you're not alone. The cholesterol readings for nearly half of American adults exceed 200 milligrams per deciliter (mg/dl) of blood, even though the National Cholesterol Education Program of the National Institutes of Health recommends keeping total cholesterol below the 200 mark. About 30 percent of us are in the borderline category, between 200 and 239 mg/dl. And almost 20 percent of us have what's defined as high cholesterol, with readings of 240 mg/dl or higher.

The good news is that while elevated cholesterol is a significant risk factor for cardiovascular trouble, it's one that's within your control. Lifestyle strategies—like watching your diet, getting regular exercise, and reducing your stress level—can lower your cholesterol reading to where it ought to be. In fact, they're often the first line of treatment recommended by physicians before prescription medications. Certain natural remedies can help, too.

If your total cholesterol is below 200, this book can help keep it there. Should it be hovering in the high or borderline range, the doctor-endorsed advice in the pages that follow can help whittle it down to a desirable level, perhaps averting the need for long-term drug therapy or surgery.

Even if you've already been diagnosed with heart disease, don't give up. Research has shown that people with severe heart disease can turn their health around. One study—the Multicenter Lifestyle Demonstration Project, led by Dean Ornish, M.D., president and director of the Preventive Medicine Research Institute in Sausalito, California—was designed to assess the effectiveness and cost efficiency of adopting heart-friendly lifestyle strategies. Candidates for bypass surgery or angioplasty were able to postpone the procedures for at least 3 years by making the sorts of changes recommended in hospital programs that adhered to Dr. Ornish's guidelines.

A previous study—the Lifestyle Heart Trial, also led by Dr. Ornish—concluded that many people with heart disease can stop and even reverse their conditions with lifestyle strategies alone. Odds are you can do it, too.

WHAT IS CHOLESTEROL, ANYWAY?

Cholesterol is a soft, waxy substance found in every human cell, in blood, and in food. The kind found in food is called dietary cholesterol. Only animal-based foods such as meat and dairy products contain dietary cholesterol; it's not found in plant-based foods such as fruits, vegetables, beans, and grains.

Believe it or not, cholesterol isn't as evil as you might think. Your body actually needs the stuff, and your cells make what they need. Your liver, for example, uses cholesterol to make bile acids, which help you digest food.

But too much cholesterol circulating in your blood can lead to trouble. One study, the Multiple Risk Factor Intervention Trial, evaluated nearly 360,000 American men, none of whom had yet experienced a heart attack. After 7 years, the investigators found that the risk of dying of coronary heart disease was two times higher in men with total cholesterol above 220 mg/dl than in men with total cholesterol of 180 mg/dl or less. Men with readings of 245 mg/dl had triple the risk.

Studies of women show that before menopause, their levels of blood cholesterol tend to average about 10 points lower than men's. At menopause, however, the gap closes, and women seem to run the same risk as men.

Cholesterol doesn't dissolve in blood, so it can't get to where the body needs it on its own. It has to hitch a ride on special carriers called lipoproteins. There are two major types: low-density lipoprotein (LDL) and high-density lipoprotein (HDL). LDL, the "bad" type, is packed with cholesterol, while HDL, the "good" cholesterol, is mostly protein.

If there's too much LDL in your blood, it gets deposited on the walls of your arteries as fatty clumps. If these clumps break free, they can cause the blood to clot. A clot that cuts off the flow of blood to the heart can cause a heart attack; a clot that blocks bloodflow to the brain can trigger a stroke.

HDL, on the other hand, is a cardiovascular hero. It patrols your arteries, hauling cholesterol away from them and carrying it to the liver for dumping. Experts agree that the higher your level of HDL, the better your cardiovascular health is likely to be. One study has concluded that for each 1 mg/dl rise in HDL, the risk of coronary heart disease declines by 2 to 3 percent.

"People are asking, 'What more can we do?' " says Daniel J. Diver, M.D., head of cardiology at Saint Francis Hospital and Medical Center in Hartford, Connecticut. The answer is to increase HDL levels. Research has shown that HDL levels are the best gauge of long-term survival in people who have undergone bypass surgery. "In the past few years," Dr. Diver says, "HDL has emerged as an independent predictor of heart disease."

Whenever you have a cholesterol test, the lab will also measure triglycerides, another blood fat implicated in coronary heart disease, since many people with high triglycerides have high LDL or low HDL levels. Triglyceride levels of less than 150 mg/dl are considered desirable.

Additionally, it's a good idea to know your level of lipoprotein (a), or Lp(a). Lp(a) is a chunk of cholesterol coated with protein, and it's found only in the blood of hedgehogs, certain monkeys—and humans. Researchers at Oxford University in England found that among people who had heart disease or who had survived a heart attack, those who had the highest levels of Lp(a) also had a 70 percent greater risk of experiencing a heart attack over a 10-year period than those with the lowest levels. Levels starting at 30 mg/dl seem to raise risk. The renowned Framingham Heart Study, which has tracked the health of the residents of Framingham, Massachusetts, for more than four decades, found that having levels of about 30 mg/dl doubled the risk of heart attack in 3,000 women. So Lp(a) tests are something to consider if you're female or you have heart disease or a family history of premature coronary artery disease or stroke.

WHY YOU SHOULD WAGE A PLAQUE ATTACK

Improving your cholesterol profile will require some effort on your part. But the payoff is well worth it. Perhaps these benefits will help fire up your resolve.

You can stay a step ahead of heart disease. In atherosclerosis (hardening of the arteries), fatty deposits called plaques stick to the walls of arteries, which channel oxygen-rich blood throughout your body. When plaques form in the arteries that supply blood to your heart, they can lead to coronary heart disease, marked by blockages in these arteries. If left untreated, the blockages can choke off your heart's blood supply, leading to chest pain (angina), heart attack, and sometimes death.

Lowering your cholesterol can reduce your chances of atherosclerosis and coronary heart disease. One landmark study, the Lipid Research Clinics Coronary Primary Prevention Trial, found that for every 1 percent reduction in total cholesterol, the probability of developing coronary heart disease or having a heart attack falls by 2 percent. The same study showed that as cholesterol levels dip, so does the incidence of angina and the need for coronary bypass surgery.

You can reduce your risk of stroke. One study found that elevated cholesterol produces abnormal amounts of a chemical that can cause spasms in the carotid artery, which is located in the neck and supplies blood to the brain. If these spasms interrupt bloodflow, they could cause a mini-stroke, or transient ischemic attack. In addition, when a plaque breaks free from an artery wall, it can cause a blood clot that blocks bloodflow to the brain, triggering a full-blown stroke.

If you have diabetes, you can head off cardiovascular complications. Some research suggests that both women and men with diabetes are about twice as likely to develop coronary heart disease as the general population. People with diabetes who have had a coronary event are twice as likely to experience repeat problems, such as angina, heart attack, and the need for bypass surgery. People with diabetes also tend to have high levels of triglycerides. If you have diabetes, lowering your cholesterol and controlling other risk factors such as high blood pressure and being overweight can cut the chances of developing diabetes-related heart and blood vessel problems.

You can increase your quantity of life. The Framingham Heart Study has shown that the lower cholesterol levels fall, the lower the chance of heart attack and sudden death becomes.

You can enhance your quality of life. Taking charge of elevated cholesterol now could mean the difference between a future of shuttling to and from the doctor's office (or the hospital) and enjoying a full, happy, healthy life.

A CORNUCOPIA OF NATURAL CHOLESTEROL "PRESCRIPTIONS"

If your cholesterol is high, one recourse is to take cholesterol-lowering drugs, which can do a great deal to keep LDL levels in check. Unfortunately, they come at a price. Since they're metabolized in the liver, you have to be monitored regularly for liver damage. So anything that can be done to lower cholesterol naturally can help minimize your doctor's need to prescribe a drug.

In the chapters that follow, you'll read about practical, expert-endorsed strategies that can help you wallop high cholesterol without the use of prescription drugs. Some of these tactics may sound familiar; others are on the cutting edge of medical research. Provided that your physician gives you the green light, you can add virtually all of these strategies to your daily routine with a minimum of time, money, and effort.

Along the way, you'll gain a wealth of practical information that can help you achieve your ultimate goal—a heart-healthy cholesterol level. You'll discover:

- Ways that olive oil, avocados, chocolate, and other indulgences can help boost your good cholesterol and lower your bad cholesterol
- Ongoing research suggesting that certain vitamins and minerals may help reduce cholesterol and protect against coronary heart disease

• A handy table of the saturated fat and cholesterol con-
tents of common foods

Think of this book as your own personal cholesterol-
reduction tool. The sooner you put it to work, the sooner
you'll reap your reward: a strong, healthy heart primed
to provide years of vibrant living.

CHAPTER TWO

The New Science of Cholesterol Control

Uncle Sam wants you . . . to guard against high cholesterol.

In 2001, the federal government's National Heart, Lung, and Blood Institute (NHLBI) issued a report declaring that healthy eating, regular exercise, and weight control are the first line of defense in the prevention and treatment of high cholesterol.

Lifestyle changes alone can help some people rein in their elevated cholesterol, particularly the "bad" LDL cholesterol, which is a major cause of coronary artery disease. But eating more vegetables and taking more brisk walks can also benefit the 13 million men and women who take cholesterol-lowering drugs, according to the authors of the report.

The institute refers to this approach as "therapeutic lifestyle changes," or TLC. This TLC concept contains four steps that lead to lower cholesterol. Following the information and advice that you'll find throughout this book will help you meet these four heart-healthy goals.

of saturated fat—the artery-clogging fat
bacon, butter, and full-fat cheese—to
t of total daily calories and limit intake
rol to no more than 200 milligrams a

- Get 10 to 25 grams of soluble fiber a day, found in
foods such as cereal grains, beans, fruits, and vegetables.
The NHLBI also encourages the use of cholesterol-
lowering margarines such as Benecol and Take Control,
which contain plant substances known as sterols and
stanols.
- Get at least 30 minutes of physical activity a day.
- Lose weight.

KNOW YOURSELF AND YOUR CHOLESTEROL

The National Cholesterol Education Program, an initia-
tive of the NHLBI, advises everyone age 20 and over to
get their cholesterol checked at least once every 5 years.
For men over 45 and women over 55, more frequent
testing may be in order, since cholesterol levels tend to
rise with age. Once you receive your results, your doctor
will likely recommend a retest if any of your numbers
are cause for concern.

The test is done on a blood sample from your finger or
arm. The resulting measurements are expressed as milligrams per deciliter (mg/dl) of blood. For a test of total
cholesterol and HDL levels, you don't need to fast before-
hand. For a complete lipid profile, which measures total
cholesterol, HDL, LDL, and triglycerides (a type of blood
fat), you must fast for 9 to 12 hours. That means no food
and no beverages except water, black coffee, or tea.

Recently, some researchers have proposed that certain

"normal" or "borderline" test res... well as for triglycerides and blood ... ally be unhealthy—and could be early ... heart disease.

To interpret your cholesterol profile, th... ... Heart Association (AHA) offers the followin... ...delines:

Total Cholesterol
Desirable: less than 200 mg/dl
Borderline: 200 to 239 mg/dl
High: 240 mg/dl or higher

If your total cholesterol is less than 200 mg/dl and you have no other risk factors, you're not very likely to develop heart disease. On the other hand, a reading in the borderline range is reason for caution. Even if you have no other risk factors, you should try to get your total cholesterol below 200 mg/dl.

If your total cholesterol falls in the high category, it's definitely a red flag for heart disease risk. You may be especially vulnerable if you have other risk factors. In this situation, your best bet is to consult your doctor about further testing and treatment options.

LDL
Optimal: less than 100 mg/dl
Above optimal: 100 to 129 mg/dl
Borderline high: 130 to 159 mg/dl
High: 160 to 189 mg/dl
Very high: 190 mg/dl or higher

If your LDL reading is in the borderline-high, high, or very high categories, your doctor will evaluate your

factors to determine whether you need to take
steps to lower it.

HDL
Desirable: 40 mg/dl or higher

On average, men have HDL in the range of 40 to 50
mg/dl; women's levels tend to be in the range of 50 to
60 mg/dl. Your doctor can interpret your readings and
tell you whether you need to take steps to raise your
HDL level.

Triglycerides
Normal: less than 150 mg/dl
Borderline high: 150 to 199 mg/dl
High: 200 to 499 mg/dl
Very high: 500 mg/dl or higher

Lifestyle changes, including diet and exercise, are the
chief strategies that doctors suggest to lower a person's
triglyceride level.

WHAT'S YOUR RATIO?

Most experts believe that your total cholesterol isn't the
most important number, since a high level of HDL—the
good kind—can drive up your cholesterol reading. Many
experts, including those at the famous Framingham Cardiovascular Institute in Massachusetts, urge patients to
focus on their levels of LDL—the bad kind—and their
ratios of total cholesterol to HDL, which may be the
most accurate gauge of heart health. The institute recommends aiming for a total cholesterol/HDL ratio of less

than 4 to 1; most experts agree that 3.5 to 1 or lower is even better.

For example, let's say that your total cholesterol is 250 mg/dl and your HDL is 50 mg/dl. Dividing 250 by 50 gives you a ratio of 5 to 1. But by cutting your total cholesterol to a nearly ideal 200 mg/dl while holding your HDL at 50 mg/dl, you'll shrink your ratio to a more desirable 4 to 1.

Doctors participating in the Physicians' Health Study—an ongoing study of more than 22,000 American doctors conducted at Harvard Medical School and Brigham and Women's Hospital in Boston—found that cutting just one unit from their ratios slashed their heart attack risk by 53 percent.

LEARNING EVEN MORE ABOUT THE SOURCE OF THE PROBLEM

Experts once thought that atherosclerosis, the buildup of cholesterol-packed plaque in arteries, was a lot like icky buildup in an old pipe. Therefore, they reasoned, controlling cholesterol could reduce heart attack risk the way a weekly dose of drain cleaner prevents clogged pipes.

Now they're realizing that their theory may have been too simplistic. According to groundbreaking research, the buildup of plaque often begins when the smooth cells lining the artery walls are injured or irritated. The culprits include LDL cholesterol that has been oxidized, or altered by renegade molecules called free radicals; homocysteine, a naturally occurring amino acid; and apolipoprotein B (apo B), a protein that carries cholesterol into artery walls.

Many of these recently discovered risk factors can be checked using new tests. While they won't replace regular cholesterol testing, they will provide valuable information about the state of your heart health. If you have other risk factors for heart disease, you may want to discuss these tests with your doctor.

Homocysteine. Having some of this amino acid in your blood is normal and apparently harmless. But more than a dozen studies suggest that slightly elevated levels—above 9 micromoles per liter—may greatly raise your risk for a heart attack or stroke, even when your cholesterol levels are normal.

The Abbott homocysteine test costs about $80, depending on your insurance carrier. Test results are available within hours.

Apolipoprotein A-1 (apo A-1) and apolipoprotein B (apo B). These two substances speed through the bloodstream carrying chunks of cholesterol. Apo A-1 rounds up potentially heart-harming fats and delivers them to the liver, while apo B carries cholesterol to artery walls and leaves it behind.

The riskiest situation is having a low level of apo A-1 and a high level of apo B. One study of 1,000 people showed that this combination quadrupled the odds of a second heart attack. It may be bad news even for people who haven't had a heart attack.

Consult your doctor about the test for apo A-1 and apo B, which costs $100 to $120.

Lipoprotein (a). No one knows the purpose of lipoprotein (a), or Lp(a), which is basically a cholesterol chunk wrapped in a protein coat. Several studies, however, including one at Oxford University in England, have established an association between a high Lp(a) level and an elevated heart disease risk.

Ask your doctor about having your Lp(a) level checked. Specialized laboratories will administer the test for about $75.

C-reactive protein (CRP). This substance is produced in the liver when arteries are inflamed. It's a kind of early-warning system, with high levels indicating whether plaque is likely to rupture. In the Harvard Physicians' Health Study, high levels of CRP predicted a first heart attack 6 to 8 years in advance and were associated with a threefold increase in risk.

Ask for the high-sensitivity CRP (hs-CRP) test, not a standard CRP test, which is used for diagnosing conditions such as arthritis and inflammatory bowel disease. The test costs $60 and is widely available.

PART II

Treatments and Remedies

CHAPTER THREE

What Your Doctor Can Do

In keeping with the latest findings about the importance of lifestyle changes in bringing down cholesterol, doctors nowadays aren't as quick to prescribe cholesterol-lowering medications for people with low to moderate risk of heart disease.

Instead, they'll instruct these patients to improve their eating habits, increase their physical activity, and shed any extra pounds they may be carrying. By themselves, this trio of strategies may be enough to whip an unhealthy cholesterol profile into shape.

But if you try these changes and they don't produce the results you need within about 6 months, your doctor may recommend using a cholesterol-lowering medication. The benefits offered by doctor-prescribed treatments can be dramatic and underscore just how lifesaving cholesterol control can be.

If you're at high risk for heart disease, your doctor has likely put you on cholesterol-lowering medication already. Adding lifestyle changes, as well as some of the other remedies in later chapters, may give you even better and faster results.

MEDICATIONS: BEATING THE ODDS FOR THOSE AT HIGH RISK

While cholesterol-lowering medications abound, three categories are most popular: statins, bile acid resins, and a form of the B vitamin niacin. All three lower LDL cholesterol, which is important because a high level of LDL has the most serious impact on heart disease risk. Niacin also lowers total cholesterol and triglycerides while raising "good" HDL cholesterol.

Statins. Some of the most widely prescribed cholesterol-lowering drugs, statins work by slowing the body's production of cholesterol and helping the liver remove LDL that's already in the blood. Studies have linked statins with 20 to 60 percent reductions in LDL, along with slight increases in HDL and declines in triglycerides.

In a Scandinavian study involving a statin, the participants experienced a 25 percent reduction in total cholesterol and a 35 percent reduction in LDL cholesterol. In turn, the death rate for the group dropped by 42 percent; the likelihood of nonfatal heart attacks, by 37 percent; and the need for heart surgery (bypass or angioplasty), by 27 percent.

Five statin drugs are currently available: lovastatin (Mevacor), simvastatin (Zocor), pravastatin (Pravachol), fluvastatin (Lescol), and atorvastatin (Lipitor). A sixth drug, cerivastatin (Baycol), was withdrawn from the market in 2001, after some people taking the medication experienced potentially serious side effects.

Once you've been taking the [...] weeks, your doctor will probably send [...] terol test, then average those results with [...] to see how the statin is working. Because y[...] produces more cholesterol at night, plan to take [...] medication in the early evening or at bedtime.

The potential side effects of statins include mild discomforts such as gas, upset stomach, constipation, and abdominal cramps. These should disappear as your body adjusts to treatment. Rarely, liver abnormalities and muscle problems can also develop.

Bile acid resins. These medications "pick up" cholesterol-containing bile acids in the intestines and carry them out of the body. This reduces LDL levels by 10 to 20 percent—or by more than 40 percent when the resins are taken in combination with statins.

Two commonly prescribed resins are cholestyramine (Prevalite) and colestipol (Colestid). Although both drugs appear safe for long-term use, they can cause gas, bloating, constipation, and nausea. Experts recommend mixing the powder form with water or fruit juice; if you're taking the tablets, wash them down with lots of water to prevent gastrointestinal side effects. Also, if you're on any other medications, take them either an hour before or 4 to 6 hours after the resins, since the resins may affect their absorption.

Niacin. In high daily doses of 1,000 to 3,000 milligrams, niacin—also known as vitamin B_3—has been shown to dramatically improve the entire cholesterol profile. In studies, it lowered LDL by 10 to 25 percent, raised HDL by 15 to 35 percent, and decreased triglycerides by 20 to 50 percent.

Niacin lowers LDL by partially blocking the release

d by limiting the liver's
ow density lipoprotein).
erted to LDL, reducing it
cline in LDL.

in over the counter, the high
erol control are available only
e that you're taking the form
e the form called nicotinamide
or niac... ffect on cholesterol.

Although a... ...ne study has linked niacin with liver abnormalities, more recent research suggests that as long as it's given in the proper dose, such complications are relatively rare. You must have your niacin usage supervised by a physician, who should monitor your liver enzymes to guard against possible serious liver side effects.

The other troublesome side effect of niacin is the flushing that most people who take it initially experience. It should subside as your body adjusts. In addition, research indicates that flushing can be eliminated in 80 percent of cases by taking niacin with meals; avoiding alcohol, spicy foods, and hot liquids; and not skipping doses. Some niacin is designed to be taken at bedtime so that any flushing occurs while you sleep.

In some people, niacin therapy triggers high blood sugar and gout. Your doctor may not prescribe niacin if you already have diabetes or high uric acid levels (which contribute to gout).

If your cholesterol level is exceptionally high, you and your doctor may want to consider combining niacin with a statin.

CHAPTER FOUR

Edible Heart Protection

Fighting cholesterol doesn't have to put a cramp on your eating style. The list of foods you should avoid or minimize while you're trying to rein in your cholesterol isn't especially lengthy (or surprising). Among the potential troublemakers are fatty meats, butter and other fatty dairy products, egg yolks, fried foods, solid fats, and saturated oils like palm oil.

On the other hand, when considering foods that help *improve* your cholesterol profile, you enjoy a wide variety of choices: fruits, vegetables, grains, and even some popular snacks you might have considered off-limits.

You'll find suggestions in this chapter on creative ways to add these to your diet. But if you really want to use many of these choices to their fullest potential, consult a low-fat cookbook for ideas, such as *Healthy Homestyle Cooking*, by Evelyn Tribole, M.S., R.D.

VEGETABLES: STOCK UP ON AVOCADOS, CARROTS, ONIONS, AND MORE

For many of us, hating vegetables was as much a part of childhood as climbing trees or playing with dolls. Fortunately, most of us outgrew this disdain. As adults, we not only acquired a taste for beans, broccoli, and bok choy, we began to appreciate their health benefits, too.

Vegetables are virtually fat-free, a boon if you're on a cholesterol-lowering program. "As you add more vegetables to your diet, you tend to consume less fat," says Martin Yadrick, R.D., a dietitian in Manhattan Beach, California, and a spokesperson for the American Dietetic Association. Vegetables are also loaded with fiber—both the insoluble kind, which promotes bowel regularity and may lessen the risk of colon cancer, and the soluble variety, which helps trounce blood cholesterol levels. Soluble fiber is found in many favorite vegetables, including peas, corn, and potatoes. (For more fiber information, see page 31.)

Best of all, veggies are so low in calories that you can eat virtually as many juicy beefsteak tomatoes, crisp snow peas, and colorful red, orange, and yellow peppers as you wish. "Americans like to eat lots of food," says Janet Lepke, R.D., a dietitian in Santa Monica, California, and a spokesperson for the American Dietetic Association. "When people eat less, they tend to feel deprived. But you can eat a lot of vegetables and feel good about it."

Some of the most compelling studies of the cholesterol-lowering benefits of vegetables—and fruits—were conducted on the other side of the world from America, in India.

In one study, researchers put more than 600 people who were at risk for coronary heart disease on a low-fat, low-cholesterol diet. Half of them were instructed to increase their intakes of fruits and vegetables to 400 or more grams (about five servings) a day; the others were not. After 12 weeks, the total cholesterol of the folks who ate the most fruits and vegetables dropped an average of 6.5 percent, and their "bad" LDL cholesterol dropped 7.3 percent. What's more, these folks' heart-healthy HDL cholesterol rose 5.6 percent. The total and LDL cholesterol of those who didn't eat the extra roughage remained the same.

In another Indian study, researchers put 400 people who had previously had heart attacks on a low-fat, low-cholesterol diet. As in the first study, half of these people were instructed to eat lots of fruits and vegetables; the other half were not. After 3 months, the total cholesterol of those who maxed out on fruits and vegetables plunged 27 points, from 226 to 199 milligrams per deciliter (mg/dl) of blood. Cholesterol readings in the control group fell, too, but less dramatically—14 points, from 229 to 215 milligrams per deciliter.

If there's any bad news to eating lots of vegetables, it's that you can cancel all of these benefits if you're in the habit of drowning them in butter, cream sauce, or cheese sauce or loading them with salt. But you don't have to do without flavor. Using herbs, spices, and condiments can transform a naked baked potato or plain green beans into veritable veggie delights. And your heart will thank you.

Let's take a look at some particular anti-cholesterol crusaders from the vegetable family (including the avocado, though technically it's a fruit).

For Maximum Benefit

How you prepare nature's harvest has a great deal to do with how much benefit you will reap. Here are some helpful hints.

- Choose fresh or frozen vegetables over canned; they taste better and contain more nutrients. If you opt for frozen, read the package to make sure the product doesn't contain added salt or fat.
- Steam rather than boil vegetables to retain most of their nutrients.
- Top baked potatoes and steamed vegetables with a blend of fat-free yogurt, garlic, a sprinkling of "light" salt, and a dash each of curry and cayenne pepper.
- At your next barbecue, pass up the ribs and grill some vegetables instead. Marinate sliced eggplant in low-sodium teriyaki sauce, ginger, and garlic, then barbecue it. Try grilling big slices of mushrooms, peppers, and zucchini, too. You can find suitable skewers or racks wherever grill accessories are sold, so food doesn't fall into the coals or burners.

Avocados

Avocados are high in monounsaturated fat, which is known to reduce LDL cholesterol. The oleic acid they contain is the same cholesterol-busting monounsaturate found in olive and canola oils.

The connection between avocados and lower blood cholesterol began with a hunch: A team of Australian researchers suspected the link and decided to test their theory. In this study, 15 women alternated between a low-fat, high-carbohydrate diet (21 percent fat calories) and an avocado-enriched diet (36 percent fat calories) in which they ate from ½ to 1½ avocados per day.

After 3 weeks on the avocado-rich diet, the women's total cholesterol fell from an average of 236 to 217 mg/dl, or 8.2 percent, compared with 4.9 percent after 3 weeks on the low-fat plan. More significant, however, HDL cholesterol didn't fall on the avocado diet, but it plummeted an average of 14 percent on the low-fat plan. As a result, the ratio of total cholesterol to HDL increased 10.4 percent when the women were on the low-fat plan but *decreased* 14.9 percent when they added avocado—a beneficial result.

Avocados contain zero dietary cholesterol, which is found only in animal-derived foods such as eggs, milk, and meats. But don't gobble avocados with abandon: 71 to 88 percent of its calories come from fat. Using one-eighth of an average avocado in a salad adds about 5 grams of fat.

Many people stud their salads with chunks of avocado or add the fruit to a sandwich. But you might try topping a baked potato with some mashed avocado, or perking up baked chicken by garnishing it with a few slices before serving.

Carrots

Carrots are rich in calcium pectate, a certain type of soluble fiber that may have special cholesterol-lowering power, according to research by Peter D. Hoagland, Ph.D., a research chemist for the USDA. Dr. Hoagland's research indicates that calcium pectate helps to bind bile acids, the substances that assist in the digestion of fats and in the transportation of cholesterol out of the body.

Many experts suggest steaming carrots to preserve their nutrients. Boiling them drains 50 percent of their beta-carotene and 90 percent of their vitamin C.

Onions

Sure, chopping onions may bring tears to your eyes or start your nose running like a leaky faucet. But those tears and sniffles might be worth it: The same compounds in onions that leave many of us helplessly weepy-eyed may also help wallop elevated blood cholesterol and bust up blood clots that can trigger a heart attack.

There's not yet *conclusive* proof that onions can help control cholesterol or prevent a heart attack. But investigators continue to be intrigued by the potential health benefits of this odoriferous bulb. In one study, researchers in India had 10 men consume 3½ ounces of butter a day, which increased their cholesterol levels. The researchers then added about 2 ounces of juice from raw onions to the men's daily servings of butter. The onion extract prevented the rise in cholesterol from the butter. It also increased the men's clot-busting activity almost 16 percent, reducing their risk of heart attacks.

Another Indian study found that cholesterol levels were lowest among people who consumed more than 600 grams of onions and 50 grams of garlic a week— and highest among people who never touched the stuff.

Researchers in the Netherlands found that antioxidant constituents called flavonoids—found in many fruits and vegetables, including onions and apples, as well as tea— reduced the risk of coronary heart disease and heart attack in elderly men, apparently by blocking the formation of clotting compounds in the blood and by interfering with the oxidation of LDL cholesterol, which leads to the buildup of plaque in the coronary arteries.

For Maximum Benefit

Many people love onions. But if you'd like to tone down their taste—or at least dry up your tears as you slice them—these tips are for you.

- Investigate sweet onions. There are several varieties of mild-tasting onions, such as Vidalia, Walla Walla, Maui, and Texas Spring Sweet.
- Don't fry onions in oil or butter. Instead, sauté them in the microwave. Place a sliced onion in a microwave-safe bowl, along with a tablespoon or two of water. Cover the bowl with a plate. Then nuke the covered bowl for 3 to 4 minutes. The onions will be as soft as if they had been sautéed in butter.

HIGH-FIBER FOODS: HELPING TO KEEP YOUR ARTERIES CLEAN

The word *fiber* makes many people immediately think of "laxative"—not exactly anyone's favorite image. But fiber's power to keep your personal plumbing running smoothly is only part of its abilities. Numerous studies suggest that fiber can help unplug your arteries, too, by scuttling elevated cholesterol.

Fiber is the part of plant foods that the body can't digest, and it passes through your system pretty much intact. As we mentioned already, it comes in two basic types: soluble and insoluble. Soluble fiber, found in foods such as oat bran, barley, dried beans, peas, and apples, seems to help control the way your body produces and eliminates cholesterol.

The Coronary Artery Risk Development in Young Adults (CARDIA) Study, a multicenter project that examined heart disease risk factors in young men and women over a period of 10 years, showed that young adults who ate at least 21 grams of fiber a day gained 8 pounds less than people who ate the same number of calories but less than 12 grams of fiber a day. Since weight control also helps cholesterol control, that adds to the benefits of fiber.

Americans consume on average only about 12 grams of fiber a day. We should be eating 25 to 30 grams per day. Fortunately, it's easy to "fiber up" your diet.

For Maximum Benefit

• To limit gas and bloating—common side effects of consuming more fiber—add fiber-rich foods to your diet slowly, says James W. Anderson, M.D., professor of medicine and clinical nutrition at the University of Kentucky College of Medicine in Lexington and author of *Dr. Anderson's High-Fiber Fitness Plan*.

• Be sure to eat the skins of fruits and vegetables, such as apples and potatoes. Also, enjoy plenty of fruits with edible seeds, such as figs and blueberries.

• Try to get your fiber from foods rather than from fiber supplements. Fiber-rich foods contain nutrients that supplements lack, says Alicia Moag-Stahlberg, a spokesperson for the American Dietetic Association. Fruits and vegetables contain antioxidant vitamins, for example, which may help prevent heart disease and cancer.

Cold Cereal

When you're in the cereal aisle, skip the sugar-coated stuff and pick up a high-fiber brand.

"Replacing a daily high-fat breakfast, such as eggs and bacon, with a breakfast of cereal high in soluble fiber with fat-free milk can lower cholesterol from 8 to 16 percent within a month," says Dr. Castelli.

Several studies have analyzed the effect of high-fiber cereal on blood cholesterol. In one study, researchers at the University of Minnesota in Minneapolis had 58 men with high cholesterol follow a low-fat, low-cholesterol diet for 6 weeks. For the next 6 weeks, the men ate the same diet, with one adjustment: They also consumed either cereal enriched with pectin or psyllium fiber, or cornflakes with no soluble fiber.

The men's total cholesterol declined about 4 percent on the low-fat diet alone. But the total cholesterol of the men who ate the low-fat diet and the pectin-enriched cereal dropped 6.4 percent, and their LDL cholesterol fell 8.4 percent. The men who consumed the psyllium-enriched cereal saw their blood fats drop even more: Their total cholesterol fell 9.2 percent, and their LDL cholesterol plummeted 9.7 percent. The total and LDL cholesterol of the cornflake-eaters didn't change.

... at least 3 grams of
... or less of fat per serving, Dr. Anderson

..., look for as whole a grain of cereal as you can
... The box should specify "whole oats," "whole bar-
...ey," or "whole millet." One brand worth trying is Kashi,
a blend of oats, long-grain brown rice, rye, barley, and
other whole grains.

Oats

Remember the oat bran craze of the late 1980s? Reacting
to several encouraging medical studies—and resulting
newspaper headlines—cholesterol-conscious people began eating oat bran by the bowlful. Food manufacturers,
reacting to our sudden enthusiasm for all things oat bran,
added it to just about everything. (Some bakeries were
even selling oat bran doughnuts!)

Then, as suddenly as it began, it seemed, the oat bran
mania died, a casualty of more headlines. This time,
news stories reported, a study had concluded that oat
bran is no better at lowering blood cholesterol than white
bread.

End of story? No. Oats do appear to cause a reduction
in blood cholesterol, and experts say that oats can be a
valuable part of a low-fat diet.

Oats contain lots of soluble fiber, the kind proven to
reduce LDL cholesterol. "When you cook oats, they're
sticky," says Kay Stanfill, R.D., adjunct assistant professor in the department of nutritional sciences at the
University of Oklahoma Health Sciences Center in
Oklahoma City. "That sticky, gelatinous matter is soluble fiber."

Barley, beans, and many fruits and vegetables also contain soluble fiber. But there is something unique about oats' cholesterol-busting ability, Dr. Anderson says. "While oat bran and beans have roughly equivalent overall cholesterol-lowering effects, oat bran preserves HDL cholesterol a little better," he says.

Researchers have conducted a number of studies on the association between consuming oat bran and lower blood cholesterol levels. Investigators at Northwestern University Medical School in Chicago divided 80 men and women with high cholesterol into two groups. The first group ate two servings (about 4 ounces total) of instant oats a day. The second group stuck to their normal eating habits. After 8 weeks, the oat group's total cholesterol had declined by about 15 mg/dl.

At the University of Kentucky College of Medicine, 20 men with high cholesterol consumed diets supplemented with either oat bran or wheat bran, both of which were added to cereal and muffins. After 3 weeks, the total cholesterol of the men eating oat bran had fallen 12.8 percent, and their LDL cholesterol had declined 12.1 percent. The men who consumed wheat bran saw no such declines in cholesterol.

In an attempt to summarize the existing research on oat bran and cholesterol, researchers from around the world pooled data from 10 studies and 1,300 people. The researchers found that people who ate 3 grams of the soluble fiber found in oat bran (equal to about 1⅓ bowls of oat bran cereal) a day saw their blood cholesterol fall an average of nearly 6 mg/dl in 3 months or less. What's more, those who began with the highest cholesterol readings (230 mg/dl or more) experienced the greatest decreases in blood cholesterol—an average decline of 16 mg/dl.

For Maximum Benefit

• Choose a whole oat product. Look for the words "rolled oats," "steel-cut oats," "Irish oats" or "oat bran." Instant oatmeal probably isn't a whole oat product.

• To make it more flavorful, top a bowl of oat bran or oatmeal with a low-fat, low-cholesterol topping such as fresh fruit or a dollop or two of fat-free yogurt.

• Mix oat bran or oatmeal into ground-meat dishes, casseroles, and pancakes.

• Be wary of store-bought oat bran muffins. "They can contain a lot of fat," says Robert J. Nicolosi, Ph.D., director of the Cardiovascular Disease Control Center at the University of Lowell in Massachusetts. "The ideal way to get fiber is through grains and cereals."

FRUITS: NOT JUST AN APPLE A DAY

When you top your breakfast cereal with strawberries or plunge your fork into a slice of watermelon, it's good news for your tastebuds—and your cholesterol level. With few exceptions, fruit is virtually fat-free. Further, fruit is packed with soluble and insoluble fiber.

"Grapefruit, apples, and strawberries are just some of the good sources of soluble fiber," says Wahida Karmally, R.D., director of nutrition at the Irving Center for Clinical Research at Columbia-Presbyterian Medical Center in New York City and a member of the American Heart Association's nutrition committee. Pears, prunes, and bananas are also good sources. Most fruits contain the soluble fiber pectin, a gummy substance that acts as a natural cholesterol cutter.

There's considerable evidence that the soluble fiber in fruits and vegetables helps suck up artery-clogging cholesterol and escort it out of the body.

Researchers at the University of Minnesota in Minneapolis and the University of California, Davis, had 41 men with mildly to moderately high cholesterol add 12 prunes a day to their regular diets. After a month, the men's total cholesterol dropped from 230 to 225 mg/dl, and their LDL cholesterol fell from 158 to 151 mg/dl.

There's another heart-healthy reason to fill up on fruit. Many varieties of fruit—particularly berries, cantaloupe, and citrus—are brimming with vitamin C, an antioxidant nutrient that some studies have linked to lower rates of heart disease. Researchers at the University of California, Los Angeles, studied more than 11,000 adults for 10 years and found that people who consumed the most vitamin C had a lower risk of dying of heart disease and a lower death rate overall than people with the lowest intakes of vitamin C.

For Maximum Benefit

• Sample the more exotic fruits that you see at the corner fruit stand or in the produce section of your supermarket. Discovering the delights of kiwifruit, passion fruit, mangoes, papayas, and fresh pineapple can make eating more fruit an adventure rather than a chore.

• If you're more the classic type, treat yourself to a classic dish: fruit salad. Slice up some melon, apples, bananas, and peaches, and top the fruit with a bit of shredded coconut—but don't overdo the coconut, since it's very high in saturated fat. Splash fruit juice over the salad to further boost the flavor.

- Stir sliced fresh strawberries or bananas into a cup of low-fat or fat-free vanilla yogurt.
- Top pancakes or waffles, prepared with a low-fat mix, with fresh fruit. Try bananas, strawberries, fresh or frozen peaches, blueberries, or even apples sautéed with a pinch of cinnamon and nutmeg.

Apples

Apples in particular can lower cholesterol in special ways. They, too, contain pectin, which cuts cholesterol by drawing it out of the body. The average apple contains 1.08 grams of pectin.

Apples also contain flavonoids, certain chemicals that seem to short-circuit the process that leads "bad" LDL cholesterol to accumulate in the bloodstream. Dutch researchers who conducted a 5-year study of 805 men ages 65 to 84 found that the men who ate the most flavonoids (also found in onions, tea, and wine) were 50 percent less likely to have a first heart attack and die of heart disease than those who consumed the least.

OILS: OLIVE AND CANOLA ARE YOUR FRIENDS

People talk about the fat content of their food a lot: A low-fat diet. Fat-free cookies. Reduced-fat snack chips. Grams of fat per serving.

Painting all fats and oils as enemies is inaccurate, however, since not all fats have the same harmful effects on your health. Tossing your healthy oil out the window along with unhealthy fatty steaks and doughnuts robs you of opportunities to lower your cholesterol and make your heart healthier. Let's look at two of the common health-promoting oils.

Olive Oil

All hail olive oil, the golden essence of the Mediterranean, the nectar of the gods, the cholesterol crusher!

This fragrant oil, touted by the great Greek physician Hippocrates as a natural remedy more than 2,000 years ago, is brimming with monounsaturated fat. One study suggests that the monounsaturated fat in olive oil may actually change the chemical composition of HDL cholesterol, making it better at routing LDL. No wonder some heart experts have recommended substituting olive oil for the artery-clogging saturated fat that plagues the typical American diet.

Not surprisingly, people in the Mediterranean region, where most olive oil is produced and enthusiastically consumed, have reaped the greatest health benefits from the oil—a phenomenon first proven by Ancel Keys, Ph.D., professor emeritus of public health in the School of Public Health at the University of Minnesota in Minneapolis.

In the Seven Countries Study, a seminal project dating back to the 1950s, Dr. Keys discovered that while Italian, Greek, and other Mediterranean men consumed almost as much dietary fat as American men, most of that fat took the form of olive oil. He associated the Mediterraneans' consumption of monounsaturated fat, particularly olive oil, with their lower rates of heart disease.

More current studies have reached similar conclusions about the cholesterol-busting powers of olive oil. Re-

AN OLIVE OIL PRIMER

When it comes to olive oil, a little goes a long way. "Compared with some other oils, olive oil is so flavorful that you can use less of it," says Barbara Levine, R.D., Ph.D., associate clinical professor of nutrition in medicine at Weill Medical College of Cornell University in New York City.

Olive oil connoisseurs categorize the flavor of olive oil as mild (with a light or buttery taste), semifruity (a stronger, more olivelike flavor), or fruity (oil with an intense olive flavor). And despite what you may have heard, the color of olive oil has nothing to do with its flavor. Like wine, olive oil gets its unique color, flavor, and aroma from the olives used and the climate and soil conditions in which they were grown. So you may want to taste-test olive oil to find the variety and brand most pleasing to your palate.

As far as the other common olive-oil terminology, according to the International Olive Oil Council, virgin olive oil is oil that's pressed from olives—not brought out with solvents—and contains no more than 2 percent oleic acid. Extra-virgin olive oil is virgin olive oil with a slightly better aroma and flavor and contains no more than 1 percent oleic acid.

Here's how to get more olive oil into your diet.

• Spread crusty bread with olive oil rather than butter. Or rub a toasted slice of bread with a piece of garlic, then drizzle the bread with olive oil.
• Dress salads the Mediterranean way—with a small amount of extra-virgin olive oil and a little bit of vinegar.
• Brush corn on the cob with extra-virgin olive oil rather than butter or margarine.
• Don't forget that olive oil is still 100 percent fat and contains 120 calories per tablespoon. So overusing olive oil may cause you to gain weight—not a heart-smart move, experts say.

searchers at the Universidad Autonoma de Madrid in Spain had 21 pre- and postmenopausal women follow a high-fat diet for 4 months. For the first month of the study, the women ate a diet high in saturated fat, such as butter, and lower in polyunsaturated and monounsaturated fats. For the next 6 weeks, the women followed an olive oil–rich diet lower in saturated and polyunsaturated fats. And for 6 weeks after that, the women consumed a diet rich in sunflower oil, a polyunsaturated fat, and lower in monounsaturated and saturated fats.

The women's total and LDL cholesterol fell on both the olive oil and sunflower oil diets. But their HDL cholesterol increased on the olive oil diet—and fell on the sunflower oil diet.

But make no mistake: Drowning your food in olive oil will not protect your heart from the ravages of ribs, french fries, and rocky road ice cream, experts say. Too much of any fat—even monounsaturated fat—can wreak havoc on your cholesterol level, not to mention your waistline.

The good news is that a little bit of olive oil yields a lot of flavor. What's more, you're likely to find that this golden oil tastes delicious on everything from corn on the cob to crusty peasant bread.

Canola Oil

This super oil, high in monounsaturated fat, can lower LDL cholesterol while it maintains or even raises HDL cholesterol.

Try substituting canola oil for butter when sautéing vegetables, making baked goods and sauces, or popping popcorn. It's not good in salad dressings, however, since it's too bland to add flavor to your fixings.

However you decide to use canola oil, keep it fresh. Oils high in monounsaturated fat tend to go bad faster than other oils. So if you haven't used up a bottle of canola oil about a month after opening it, store it in the refrigerator.

FISH: REEL IN THESE CHOLESTEROL CRUSHERS

If you sometimes feel as though you're swimming up-stream in the fight to lower your blood cholesterol, fish can help you turn the tide. Not only is fish low in sat-urated fat, but it also contains oils called omega-3 fatty acids, which are highly polyunsaturated fats that can work small miracles in your body. In most studies, omega-3s lowered the subjects' high cholesterol concentrations to healthier levels.

"Omega-3s appear to decrease blood levels of VLDL (very low density lipoprotein), which is manufactured by the liver," says Peter O. Kwiterovich Jr., M.D., director of the Lipid Research and Atherosclerosis Unit at Johns Hopkins University School of Medicine in Baltimore and author of *The Johns Hopkins Complete Guide for Preventing and Reversing Heart Disease*. As VLDL measurements plummet, so may blood cholesterol levels and triglycerides, another blood fat implicated in heart disease. The two most common omega-3 fatty acids are eicosapentaenoic acid (EPA) and docosahexaenoic acid (DHA).

Omega-3 fatty acids also appear to help lower blood pressure, a significant risk factor for heart attack and stroke. Moreover, omega-3s help keep blood platelets from clinging to one another, which can defend against blood clots that may trigger a heart attack or stroke.

Generally speaking, the fattier the fish is, the more omega-3 fatty acids it contains, says Margo Denke, M.D., associate professor of medicine in the Center for Human Nutrition at the University of Texas Southwestern Medical Center at Dallas. Interestingly, fish don't manufacture omega-3s. They derive these fats from ocean foods such as saltwater algae and other cold-water vegetation. "So cold-water trout, salmon, and mackerel are good sources of omega-3s, while farm-raised catfish isn't," says Dr. Denke. Other fish rich in omega-3 fatty acids include herring and bluefin tuna.

But fish has even more going for it than the cholesterol-clobbering omega-3s. Depending on the way it's prepared, fish is also lower in dietary fat than red meat or even poultry. Three ounces of broiled or baked cod, for example, contains 89 calories, 47 grams of cholesterol, and less than 1 gram of fat.

To reap all the health benefits of omega-3s, most doctors suggest that we eat fish two or three times a week. But they're less certain of how much fish we should eat. "There's no clear evidence that we need a specific amount of fish oil in our diets," Dr. Denke says. But it's best to follow an overall cholesterol-lowering diet that includes plenty of fresh fruits and vegetables, grains, and low-fat dairy products as well as fish, lean meat, and poultry.

For Maximum Benefit

• Stock up on canned tuna or salmon—it's an easy, inexpensive way to consume omega-3s. To save on calories, buy fish that's packed in water rather than oil.

• If you're buying whole fresh fish, look for clean, tight scales; bright, clear eyes (rather than cloudy or sunken); and red or pink gills. The flesh should also spring back into place when touched. Fish should have a clean smell, not a strong odor, and the surface of the fish should be moist, but not slimy.

• The healthiest ways to prepare fish include broiling, baking, grilling, and steaming. Or "oven-fry" fish. Coat the fish in egg whites—no yolks—and bread crumbs, then bake until crispy. Squeeze some lemon or orange juice over the fish and sprinkle on some dill.

SOY FOODS: DISCOVER THE JOY OF SOY

What a difference a few decades make! Once disdained as bland fare strictly for health nuts, products like soy milk, soy hot dogs, and veggie burgers have entered the mainstream. And not a moment too soon, it seems.

Scientists studying the potential healing properties of soy have discovered a grab bag of health benefits. There's evidence that adding just a small amount of soy to your diet can help fight certain cancers, soothe menopausal symptoms, boost your immune system, and, yes, lower blood cholesterol.

In October 1999, the FDA authorized that health claims associating soy protein with the reduced risk of coronary heart disease could be made on food labels. Several studies indicate that a total daily intake of 25 grams of soy protein (for example, the amount in ½ cup of Nutlettes cereal or 8 ounces of plain soy milk) as part of a low-fat diet significantly lowers total cholesterol and LDL cholesterol levels. Soybeans are a rich source of isoflavones, a class of phytoestrogens found predominantly in legumes and beans.

People in Asian countries, who tend to consume soy-rich diets, seem to have reaped many of soy's potential health benefits. The Japanese, for example, live longer than any other nationality in the world. What's more, Japanese men have the lowest rate of death from heart disease in the world, and Japanese women have the second lowest. The average Japanese person eats 50 to 80 grams (about 2 to 3 ounces) of soy food a day; the typical American eats 5 grams a day.

Why does soy send cholesterol south? Experts aren't sure. One likely reason is that soy foods, while moderately high in fat, are still lower in fat—particularly artery-choking saturated fat—than meat and dairy products. So replacing animal protein with protein from soy products would theoretically lower blood cholesterol. Soybeans also are fairly high in fiber.

There are other theories, too. Some investigators speculate that a certain substance in soy, genistein, may help keep fatty plaques from clogging the arteries. Like isoflavones, genistein is a phytoestrogen, a plant substance that some researchers believe may help prevent certain types of cancer.

Other research suggests that soy may help the liver secrete cholesterol-rich bile acids, which aid in digestion. When the liver replaces these acids, it draws from the cholesterol circulating in the blood. Presto—your blood cholesterol sinks.

Keep in mind, though, that wolfing down tofu or soy-based breakfast "sausage" on top of a burgers-and-fries diet isn't likely to reduce your cholesterol. It works only as part of a low-fat, low-cholesterol diet. And according to experts, replacing a portion of the meat and dairy foods in your diet with their tasty soy impersonators can be a heart-smart move.

For Maximum Benefit

• Look for soy-based products, from tofu and tempeh (often found in the produce section) to commercially prepared "meat products" such as vegetable burgers in your local supermarket.
• Mix mashed tofu with diced vegetables, herbs, and spices and use it as a vegetable dip or sandwich filling.
• Add cubed tofu to stir-fried vegetables.
• Crumble tofu into spaghetti sauce or chili.
• Pour soy milk over cereal or substitute it for whole milk in soups, cakes, puddings, and other dishes.

MUSHROOMS: YOU CAN FIGHT CHOLESTEROL WITH FUNGUS

You may not have thought that mushrooms could contain cholesterol-cutting powers. That's understandable; after all, these edible fungi are about 90 percent water. But the remaining 10 percent contains a mother lode of nutrients, including potassium, calcium, riboflavin, niacin, and iron.

Since the late 1960s, researchers at the National Institute of Nutrition in Tokyo have conducted tests on the effectiveness of shiitake mushrooms on blood cholesterol. In one study, researchers had young women eat 90 grams of fresh shiitake mushrooms (about five mushrooms) a day. Their average cholesterol level declined

12 percent in a week. When researchers conducted a similar experiment with 30 people over age 60, cholesterol levels fell 9 percent in a week.

What's more, mushrooms also contain phytochemicals, or plant substances that may help fight disease, according to Robert Beelman, Ph.D., professor of food science at Pennsylvania State University in University Park. Also, some mushrooms are rich in protein and contain all of the essential amino acids. Essential amino acids, which are necessary for life, can't be manufactured by our bodies; we have to obtain them from food.

While the jury is still out on mushrooms' power to lower cholesterol, these earthy-tasting vegetables can enliven almost any dish, from casseroles to stir-fries.

For Maximum Benefit

• Avoid wild mushrooms. Some types can cause liver damage or even death.

• Select mushrooms with smooth, unblemished caps, because they're the freshest.

• Toss sautéed mushrooms with white or brown rice. And forgo the butter or margarine: You can sauté 3 to 4 cups of mushrooms in a teaspoon of oil in a nonstick skillet on medium heat.

• Add shiitake mushrooms to stews, vegetable dishes, or pasta.

• Use sautéed mushrooms as a topping for chicken.

NUTS: SMALL BUT POWERFUL SNACKS

Researchers at Loma Linda University in California examined the link between eating nuts—including al-

monds, walnuts, and peanuts—and a reduced risk of
heart disease in more than 31,000 Seventh-Day Advent-
ists. The researchers found that those who ate nuts more
than four times a week had about half the risk of suf-
fering a heart attack (fatal or nonfatal) as those who ate
nuts less than once a week. Twenty-nine percent of the
nuts consumed were almonds.

If you rarely stop in the nut section of your supermarket because you're afraid of the fat content in these
natural snacks, you may be pleasantly surprised to learn
how they can help your health.

Almonds

Almonds are more than just delicious. These nuts are
loaded with calcium, which keeps bones and teeth
strong; vitamin E, an antioxidant vitamin thought to reduce the risk of heart disease and certain types of cancer;
and magnesium, which helps regulate blood pressure.

Almonds, and nuts in general, are also high in monounsaturated fat, which has been shown to lower total and
LDL cholesterol without detrimentally affecting HDL
cholesterol. Nearly two-thirds (65 percent) of the total
fat of almonds is monounsaturated.

"There are several possible reasons why almonds and
other nuts seem to be capable of lowering blood cholesterol levels," says Gary E. Fraser, M.D., Ph.D., professor
of medicine at Loma Linda University School of Public
Health. "Almost certainly, nuts' high level of monounsaturated fat is a major factor. But nuts are also a very
good source of an amino acid called arginine, which is
a dietary precursor of a chemical called nitric oxide."
This chemical, which is released in the lining of the ar-

tery wall, seems to help prevent atherosclerosis, explains Dr. Fraser.

Grabbing a fistful of raw, unsalted almonds for a snack is one way of taking advantage of their cholesterol-lowering power. But you can also try sprinkling slivered almonds on cereal, waffles, pancakes, and salads.

Walnuts

In the early days of Rome, walnuts were considered a food fit for the gods and were named *Juglans regia* in honor of Jupiter. Not a bad endorsement. These days, however, we're more likely to bemoan the walnut's high content of fat and calories than to treat ourselves to this divinely delicious nut.

It's true that an ounce of walnuts contains about 180 calories and 17 grams of fat. But hold on: Eaten in moderation, walnuts may actually help lower your blood cholesterol without sabotaging your waistline.

How can the fat-laden walnut whittle down cholesterol? The answer lies in the type of fat this nut contains. Seventy percent of the fat in walnuts is polyunsaturated, which is gentler on your heart than the artery-plugging saturated fat found in red meat, cheese, and butter. In fact, one study of the walnut notes that this nut's ratio of polyunsaturated to saturated fat is 7 to 1—"one of the highest among naturally occurring foods," the study states.

Walnuts are also rich in linolenic acid. This omega-3 fatty acid, also found in canola oil, is similar to the cholesterol-lowering omega-3s found in fatty fish.

Translation: Eat walnuts in place of, not in addition to, other fats—especially saturated fats.

For Maximum Benefit

• Sprinkle chopped shelled walnuts over steamed Brussels sprouts or baked sweet potatoes.
• Toss a small amount of chopped walnuts onto a salad. The nuts will add flavor, texture, and vitamin E.
• Add chopped walnuts to pancake batter. Use about ¼ cup of walnuts in a recipe that yields about eight 3-inch pancakes. To further reduce fat and cholesterol, prepare the batter with fat-free milk and egg substitute.

HERBS: ADDING FLAVOR AND FIGHTING CHOLESTEROL TO BOOT

Not only can you turn to food to combat cholesterol, but you can use certain herbs to give your favorite dishes even more cholesterol-clobbering punch.

Chile Peppers

For some thrill-seeking folks, eating chile peppers is as exhilarating as skydiving or rock climbing. Eyes and noses streaming, these self-proclaimed fire-eaters—who call riding the wave of chile heat "mouth surfing"—enjoy setting their tongues ablaze. And they never seem to run out of ways to send their mouths into meltdown, adding their favorite peppers to soups, stews, salsas, and sauces; roasting them and stuffing them with cheese; and even adding them to ice cream.

But those with flame-resistant gullets may actually

reap some health benefits from chile peppers. Capsaicin—the substance that gives chile peppers their bite—may also help lower triglycerides. Chile peppers may even reduce the risk of heart attack and stroke by helping break up dangerous clots in the blood.

The few studies that have explored the connection between capsaicin and blood fats have yielded intriguing results. For example, when researchers in India fed capsaicin to laboratory rats along with their normal diet, the rodents' triglyceride levels fell, although their cholesterol levels weren't affected. Researchers at the Ohio State University College of Medicine and Public Health in Columbus also administered capsaicin to rats; these rodents' triglycerides fell as well.

For Maximum Benefit

• Spice up a salad with a small amount of chile peppers, suggests Dave DeWitt, author of *The Whole Chile Pepper Book*. If you're using dried chiles, be aware that they tend to be hotter than fresh peppers.

• Mix a tiny bit of chopped chile peppers into mayonnaise or salad dressing, suggests dietitian Nancy Gerlach, R.D., food editor of *Chile Pepper Magazine*. Or add cayenne or any type of ground chile pepper to barbecue sauce. "But bear in mind that capsaicin is soluble in oil," she notes. Translation: The longer chile peppers sit in mayonnaise or salad dressing, Gerlach says, the hotter these condiments will get. So skimp on the amount of chile you use, at least at first.

• Add chile peppers to your homemade chili. "Both the type and amount of chile peppers you use are matters of personal preference," DeWitt says. "Some people use a

SMALL PEPPERS PACK BIG HEAT

There are more than 100 kinds of chile peppers, and they're available in a variety of forms, including fresh, dried, and powdered. But when it comes to generating heat, not all chiles are created equal.

You can't always judge a chile pepper's heat by its size or color. Generally speaking, the smaller the pepper, the hotter it is: Small, narrow chile peppers, including the cayenne and serrano, pack more capsaicin than larger, milder peppers, such as the poblano and Anaheim.

The jalapeño pepper is one of the most popular chiles in the United States. But while most people consider this plump, bright red or dark green pepper a real stinger, its heat pales in comparison with that of the habañero, the most blistering chile of all.

"It's the hottest pepper on record," says Dave DeWitt, author of *The Whole Chile Pepper Book.* A measurement called the Scoville unit is used to determine the heat of chile peppers, he explains. While the jalapeño pepper averages about 5,000 Scoville units, "a habañero can measure 500,000 Scoville units—100 times hotter than a jalapeño!" says DeWitt.

Chile connoisseurs say that the habañero's fire is short-lived. But when your mouth is on fire, a minute or two can seem like an eternity, so try this pepper at your own risk.

base of green chile peppers. Others prefer red." Let your tastebuds be your guide. It's simpler to add chile heat to a dish than to subtract it. "So add the chile peppers carefully and taste as you go," he cautions. "It's easy to make the food literally too hot to eat."

• Add fresh or powdered chile peppers to your favorite bread recipe, suggests Gerlach, who uses both chopped green chiles and red chile powder in her homemade loaves. "Chiles give bread a real bite," she says.

• Chile peppers can burn more than your mouth—they can scorch your skin, too. So after you handle chiles,

wash your hands with soap and water before you touch
your eyes or face. Better yet, wear gloves while chopping
chiles, especially if you have a cut on your hand or finger.
Also, avoid inhaling the peppers' fiery fumes: "The capsaicin can burn your eyes and lips," Gerlach says.

• If, despite your best efforts, eating a fiery chile pepper
dish leaves you screaming for relief, don't gulp water—
that will spread the capsaicin throughout your mouth,
DeWitt says. Rather, drink a glass of milk or eat a few
spoonfuls of yogurt. Milk contains a protein called casein
that can help smother capsaicin's flames. Rice, bananas,
and bread may douse the flames, too.

Garlic

If you're fond of garlic-laden pasta or other dishes prepared with this aromatic member of the onion family,
you're automatically paving the way toward good heart
health. Numerous studies indicate that garlic may help
overpower high cholesterol levels.

Garlic contains allicin, a compound that is activated
when the bulb is cut, crushed, or cooked. When allicin,
which contains sulfur, reacts with oxygen, it breaks
down into other compounds that give garlic its distinc-
tive odor and, medical experts speculate, provide its ap-
parent cholesterol-busting abilities.

In a European study, 40 patients with high cholesterol
consumed either 900 milligrams of garlic powder or an
inactive placebo every day for 16 weeks. The total cholesterol of the garlic powder group fell an average of 21
percent, and their triglycerides fell 24 percent. The total
cholesterol of those taking the placebo declined only 3
percent, while their triglycerides fell 5 percent.

At Tagore Medical College in India, 222 people who had had one heart attack consumed 6 to 10 grams of garlic (two to three cloves) every day for 3 or more years. Another group of 210 people took a placebo. Not only did the garlic-eaters' cholesterol levels fall an average of 9 percent, their risk of dying or of having a second heart attack declined as well. The cholesterol levels of those taking the placebo didn't change.

Experts aren't certain how much garlic might put the kibosh on cholesterol levels. One study conducted in the Netherlands concluded that it would take 7 to 28 cloves of garlic a day to help curb cholesterol. Fortunately, a more recent study conducted in the United States indicates that significantly smaller doses of garlic may do some good.

At New York Medical College in Valhalla, Stephen Warshafsky, M.D., and his colleagues in the Section of General Internal Medicine pooled data from five top studies, involving more than 400 people, of garlic's effects on cholesterol levels. According to Dr. Warshafsky's analysis of the data, one-half to one clove of garlic a day appears to lower blood cholesterol an average of 9 percent.

Aside from its cholesterol-lowering properties, garlic appears to keep blood platelets from clumping together, preventing clots that could trigger a heart attack or stroke. Garlic may also stimulate the blood's natural clot-dissolving processes, which helps get rid of clots that do form.

A word of caution, however: Since garlic has been shown to delay blood-clotting time, consult your doctor before consuming garlic or garlic supplements if you're taking blood-thinning drugs, advises Herbert Pierson,

Ph.D., vice president of Preventive Nutrition Consultants in Woodinville, Wisconsin, and former project director of the Cancer Preventive Designer Food Project at the National Cancer Institute.

For Maximum Benefit

• "One of the easiest ways to use garlic is to chop it up, crush it, and sauté it in a little olive or canola oil," says Dr. Pierson. "Then you can add it to soups, stews, and many other dishes that would benefit from the flavor of garlic."

• Add ground fresh garlic to salad dressings and marinades, suggests Mary Donkersloot, R.D., a dietitian in Beverly Hills, California, and author of *The Fast Food Diet.*

• If you'd rather not handle fresh garlic, opt for commercially prepared garlic paste or minced garlic in oil. You might also try garlic powder (made from dehydrated and pulverized cloves), garlic oil (distilled from cloves), or aged garlic extract (a water-based garlic product). One large garlic clove is equal to 1/2 teaspoon of garlic powder or 1 teaspoon of minced garlic.

• Store commercially prepared minced garlic in oil in the refrigerator and garlic powder in a cool, dark cabinet.

• Add garlic to your orange juice. Yes, you read right. "Add an odor-modified substance such as aged garlic extract to orange juice," Dr. Pierson says. "The juice tends to cover up even the slightest garlicky odor." His recipe: Blend three 8-ounce glasses of orange juice, an orange, and 1 tablespoon of aged garlic extract liquid.

• Don't use garlic salt. This product can be loaded with sodium, which is associated with a rise in blood pressure.

What's more, garlic salt doesn't possess the health benefits of fresh garlic.

• Consumed in large amounts, garlic can cause a variety of side effects, including heartburn, gas, skin irritation, and, rarely, allergic reactions in sensitive people. If you experience garlic-induced discomfort, reduce the amount of garlic you're consuming, Dr. Pierson advises. Or try cooking fresh garlic instead of eating it raw. Cooking garlic tends to weaken its irritating properties, he says.

SNACK FOODS: CHOCOLATE AND POPCORN AREN'T ALWAYS SO BAD

If you've been put on a heart-healthy diet, you may expect that your favorite snacks will become off-limits. But that's not necessarily so. If you exercise moderation, you can still bask in the glow of delicious chocolate or munch on popcorn in front of the TV without jeopardizing your cholesterol levels. Here's how.

Chocolate

Chocolate has gotten a bad rap: Too many calories, too much fat, and often, just too darned easy to overindulge in. Now there's sweeter news about chocolate. Research suggests that it not only doesn't raise levels of LDL cholesterol, it also increases HDL cholesterol. The flavonoids found in chocolate may act as antioxidants, which are thought to neutralize the artery-clogging plaque that leads to a heart attack.

Researchers at Pennsylvania State University in University Park found that eating moderate amounts of chocolate as part of an overall healthy diet may indeed help your heart.

Just remember to think of chocolate as a fun, occasional part of a balanced diet. Its new image as a heart helper doesn't mean that you can have it with breakfast, lunch, and dinner. It does contain fat, and too much of that leads to higher cholesterol and weight gain.

Also, opt for the dark stuff. Dark chocolate is made with more cocoa than milk chocolate, and premium dark chocolate has even more. While that's not a guarantee of higher levels of antioxidants, you will get an edge from lower amounts of saturated fat.

Popcorn

That ping-ping-ping of kernels inside a saucepan, air popper, or microwaveable bag will be heard billions of times in the United States this year. In an average year, we eat 18 billion quarts of popcorn!

Prepared in a heart-healthy manner, popcorn is a perfect antidote to a snack attack. "It's a high-carbohydrate, low-calorie, and filling snack," says Karen Vartan, R.D., a dietitian in Chicago. What's more, half of the fiber in popcorn is soluble, the kind that can help knock points off your blood cholesterol level.

But popcorn is only as healthful as the way it's prepared. "Air-popped popcorn is the way to go," advises Lisa Lauri, R.D., nutrition consultant at North Shore University Hospital in Manhasset, New York. A typical serving (3 cups) of air-popped popcorn contains 81 calories and just a trace of fat. Popcorn popped in oil and drenched in butter or margarine and salt, on the other hand, contains large amounts of total and saturated fat and sodium. So do many varieties of microwaveable and prepopped, ready-to-eat popcorn.

But more than a few of us believe that unless popcorn is bathed in butter and soaked with salt . . . well, it's just not popcorn. "There are two kinds of popcorn-eaters," says Vartan. "The first kind thinks that air-popped popcorn with nothing on it tastes perfectly acceptable. The second kind eats popcorn as a pleasure food, complete with butter or even chocolate. This kind of popcorn is as much a treat as premium ice cream." While there's nothing wrong with treating yourself to gourmet popcorn occasionally, says Vartan, indulging too often can help launch your intake of artery-clogging fat into orbit.

For Maximum Benefit

- To add pizzazz to air-popped corn, lightly spray it with a vegetable oil cooking spray, such as Pam, and get creative with the seasonings. Sprinkle the popcorn with some low-fat cheese—perhaps low-fat Cheddar, Monterey Jack, or Swiss—along with some caraway or mustard seeds. Other options? Try sprinkling popcorn with Butter Buds, oregano, basil, or sage.
- If you buy microwaveable or ready-to-eat popcorn, opt for "light" varieties; they contain less fat and sodium. Many brands, including Orville Redenbacher's, Jolly Time, and Pop-Secret, offer lower-fat products as well as their regular lines. Light popcorn isn't necessarily low-fat, however, so check the label for grams of fat and the percentage of calories from fat.

BEVERAGES: CONQUER CHOLESTEROL WITH WINE, TEA, JUICE, AND MILK

We've looked at a shopping basket's worth of foods that can help you lower cholesterol. Now let's look at their

PASS ON MOVIE POPCORN

If you're like a lot of people, watching the latest block-buster without a big tub of buttered popcorn is just about unthinkable. But a few years ago, a study conducted by the Center for Science in the Public Interest (CSPI) painted a picture of movie popcorn more frightening than the latest version of *Jurassic Park*.

The CSPI study found that a large tub of butter-flavored popcorn popped in coconut oil, which is 86 percent saturated fat, contains more than 1,600 calories and nearly 130 grams of fat. That's as much fat as in eight Big Macs! Even a small tub (about 5 cups) of butter-flavored popcorn popped in coconut oil packs about 20 grams of fat total, 14 of them saturated.

The good news is that more and more movie chains are offering air-popped corn or are popping popcorn in canola oil. This unsaturated fat is easier on your coronary arteries than the more commonly used coconut oil, a highly saturated fat.

Why do most theaters use coconut oil? People seem to prefer it. Also, coconut oil has a longer shelf life than unsaturated fats such as canola and corn oils, which may make coconut oil a more attractive choice to theater owners.

To avoid movie popcorn's saturated-fat attack, consider taking your own air-popped corn to the theater. You might also suggest to the manager that the theater offer air-popped corn as well as the oil-popped kind.

counterparts—the *beverages* that can help you even more.

Wine

Imagine living in Paris, where the bread is fresh, the Brie is creamy, and the croissants are butter-soaked. Nevertheless, like other French men and women, your heart

attack risk is less than half that of your American counterparts.

Welcome to the French paradox.

This phrase refers to the mysterious fact that in some
regions of France, people consume high-fat diets bursting with artery-clogging saturated fat and have high
blood cholesterol, high blood pressure, and smoking
habits similar to those of Americans—yet these folks
have lower rates of coronary heart disease. Why do the
French seem to get away with indulging in less-than-
perfect health habits?

Many researchers believe that it may in part be the
amount of wine the French consume. Studies here and
abroad have found that people who consume moderate
amounts of alcohol (even just one drink a day), as the
French tend to do, have lower rates of coronary heart
disease.

Researchers analyzing data from 17 countries, including France, noted that people in Toulouse, France, consume about 38 grams of alcohol per day (34 grams of it
as wine), compared with a much lower intake in Stanford, California. Further, the death rate from heart disease is 57 percent lower among men in Toulouse than
among men in Stanford. But the researchers noted that
alcohol "is a drug that, studies suggest, should be used
regularly but only at moderate doses of about 20 to 30
grams per day." At this level of consumption, the researchers said, "the risk of coronary heart disease can be
decreased by as much as 40 percent."

Drinking wine and other alcoholic beverages may also
boost levels of tissue-type plasminogen activator, or tPA.
This substance, found naturally in the body, helps keep
blood from clotting. In a study of more than 600 men,

THINK BEFORE YOU DRINK
**A bottle of Bordeaux won't work magic on clogged ar-
teries, says William P. Castelli, M.D., medical director
of the Framingham Cardiovascular Institute, a wellness
program at Metro West Medical Center in Massachusetts.**

And some experts feel that wine shouldn't be touted as a cholesterol buster at all. One study concluded that "the protective
effects of alcohol come at the cost of life-shortening alcohol abuse
by large numbers of people."

The bottom line? If you don't drink, don't start, says Frederic
Pashkow, M.D., a cardiologist at the Cleveland Clinic Foundation
in Ohio and author of *50 Essential Things to Do When the Doctor
Says It's Heart Disease*. "There are other ways besides drinking to
improve your cholesterol profile, including reducing the fat in your
diet and getting regular exercise," he says. "Nevertheless, if you're
already having a drink a day, and your doctor says it's okay, then
it's fine to continue to drink in moderation."

those who reported drinking two or more alcoholic beverages a day had 35 percent more tPA in their blood
than men who said they rarely or never drank.

A study by researchers at Harvard University and
Brigham and Women's Hospital in Boston examined the
relationship between heart attack (myocardial infarction)
and the type of alcoholic beverages consumed. Study
participants who drank, on average, one-half to one or
more alcoholic beverages a day had a lower risk of heart
attack than nondrinkers. Levels of HDL were significantly higher in drinkers of all beverage categories than
in nondrinkers. The researchers credited the protective
effect of alcohol, in large part, to the increased HDL.
They suggested that regular consumption of small to
moderate amounts of alcoholic beverages, regardless of

the type, reduces the risk of myocardial infarction.

Other researchers theorize, however, that it's the antioxidants in wine, not the alcohol, that cause the beneficial effect. Some studies have shown that red wine has a potent antioxidative capacity and has reduced the oxidation of LDL cholesterol in laboratory test tubes. (Oxidation is a chemical process that appears to increase the likelihood of LDL cholesterol collecting in the arteries.) Red wine's antioxidant compounds may also hinder the buildup of fatty deposits in the coronary arteries, says John D. Folts, Ph.D., director of the University of Wisconsin Coronary Artery Thrombosis Research and Prevention Lab at the University of Wisconsin Hospital and Clinics in Madison.

If you drink, be sure to keep it in moderation (no more than two 5-ounce glasses of wine a day for men or one for women). And if you're a teetotaler, don't start drinking just to protect your health. (See chapter 11 for more information.)

Tea

If your day isn't complete without a cup or two of tea, you could be doing your heart a favor. Research indicates that tea, especially green tea, may help ward off heart disease and reduce blood cholesterol levels.

Tea is the most widely consumed beverage in the world, second only to water. The United States ranks seventh in tea consumption, behind countries such as India and Russia.

Tea leaves are processed in a variety of ways to make three basic types of tea: black, green, and oolong. Black tea, the kind that most Americans drink, is fermented—

that is, the leaves are partially dried, crushed, allowed to sit for a few hours, and then completely dried. Green tea, the variety most often consumed in Japan, Korea, and China, is simply steamed, rolled, and crushed. Oolong tea, which is partially fermented, is a cross between black and green tea. One cup of tea contains about 27 milligrams of caffeine, about one-third of the amount found in a cup of ground or roasted coffee.

It's green tea that has garnered the most scientific scrutiny—and, according to some experts, it may have the most health benefits.

Many researchers credit compounds called polyphenols for tea's cardiovascular protection. Polyphenols act as antioxidants, chemicals that help gobble up free radicals—the cell-damaging molecules thought to accelerate aging and play a role in degenerative conditions such as heart disease and cancer. Green tea is bursting with polyphenols. The fermentation process tends to alter or destroy the polyphenols in black and oolong teas, however.

Polyphenols may help hinder the oxidation of LDL cholesterol, says Dr. Nicolosi. Oxidation is the chemical process that rusts metal and turns bananas brown and spotty, and it also makes LDL particles more likely to cling to artery walls.

"Polyphenols are reported to be much more active as antioxidants than vitamin E, for example," he says. And one study suggests that the antioxidant properties in tea might help prevent blood from clotting, which can reduce the risk of heart attacks.

Tea also contains flavonoids, antioxidant compounds that seem to short-circuit the process that leads LDL cholesterol to accumulate in the bloodstream. Dutch researchers who conducted a 5-year study of 805 men ages 65 to 84 found that the men who ate the most flavonoids (also found in onions, apples, and wine) were 50 percent less likely to have a first heart attack and die of heart disease than those who consumed the least.

Two other studies have found an association between green tea consumption and cholesterol reduction.

Japanese researchers investigated the link between green tea and cardiovascular and liver diseases in 1,371 men over age 40. The researchers found that as tea consumption rose, HDL cholesterol increased, while levels of triglycerides, total cholesterol, and LDL cholesterol fell. In fact, total cholesterol in the men who drank 10 or more cups of tea a day was about 6 percent less than in the men who drank 3 or fewer cups a day.

In another Japanese study of 1,300 men, researchers found that the greater the consumption of green tea, the lower the men's cholesterol. Men who drank 2 or fewer cups of tea a day had total cholesterol levels averaging 193 mg/dl. Those who drank between 6 and 8 cups a day had an average cholesterol reading of 188 mg/dl. And the average cholesterol of men who drank 9 or more cups a day was even lower—185 mg/dl.

For Maximum Benefit

• Since there is not yet conclusive proof that tea can lower cholesterol, it's difficult to know how much tea might do the trick. Some evidence suggests that drinking a few cups of tea a day may give you a slight edge, however. If you enjoy black tea, avoid adding cream, half-and-half or whole milk, because all are high in fat. Use fat-free or low-fat milk instead.
• Most people drink green tea without cream or sugar.

You can find green tea in some large supermarkets and most health food stores and Asian groceries.

• Consume tea in moderation, especially if you're at risk for certain irregular heart rhythms, or arrhythmias. "Caffeine is a stimulant and has a tendency to accelerate the heart rate," says Connie Diekman, R.D., a dietitian in St. Louis and a spokesperson for the American Dietetic Association. People taking medication to control tachycardia, for example, may want to avoid caffeine.

Juice

According to one study, grape juice may have the ability to boost HDL cholesterol and reduce the risk of coronary heart disease as wine does. While more study is needed, grape juice could be the heart-smart teetotaler's beverage of choice.

It appears to take three times as much grape juice by volume to reap red wine's preventive benefits, says Dr. Folts. "Our studies have determined that there's a measurable antiplatelet inhibition from two glasses of red wine," he says. "It would probably take six glasses of grape juice to achieve the same effect."

Orange juice is another good bet. According to researchers at the University of Western Ontario in London, Ontario, one of the easiest things you can to do lower your cholesterol is to drink some OJ every day.

After sipping first one, then two, then three glasses of orange juice a day for 4 weeks, 25 men and women with relatively high cholesterol levels benefited in two ways: Their HDL cholesterol levels shot up 21 percent, and their LDL cholesterol levels dropped 16 percent.

"We're not completely sure why orange juice raised

HDL," says Elzbieta Kurowska, Ph.D., the study's lead author and research associate at the University of Western Ontario. "But we know that it contains hesperidin, a flavonoid less common in other citrus fruits."

The study was small, and there's a possible delay in the effect of the juice, so it's hard to say how many glasses to drink each day. "People with high total cholesterol and low HDL cholesterol could try more orange juice in their diets to see whether it improves their cholesterol profiles," Dr. Kurowska advises. (While eating whole oranges has other benefits, it's not a practical way to try to lower your cholesterol, since it takes about four medium oranges to make one glass of juice.)

Since orange juice is high in calories (110 per 8 ounces), study participants were advised to eat less of other foods to compensate. To reap the potential benefits without adding excess calories, split your daily ration of OJ by mixing 4 ounces with seltzer for midmorning and midafternoon pick-me-ups.

Fat-Free Milk

On an airplane flight, dietitian Martin Yadrick asked the flight attendant if he could have some fat-free milk. She said, "No, not unless you order a special meal. But who can drink that stuff anyway? You may as well not drink milk at all!"

If that's the way you feel about fat-free milk, you're not alone. Many an adult, contemplating the switch from whole milk to fat-free, may feel like a kid who has just watched Mom heap broccoli on his plate.

Whole milk is a good source of calcium, which helps prevent osteoporosis, and is rich in protein, minerals, and vitamins A and D. But if you're trying to lower your blood cholesterol, whole milk *doesn't* do a body good. One cup of whole milk contains 8 grams of fat, 33 milligrams of cholesterol, and 150 calories. One study concluded that Americans' passion for whole milk and whole milk products such as cheese "probably contributes substantially to the population burden of coronary heart disease."

Milk that's merely low in fat isn't the answer either. Gulping down glasses of low-fat milk, which contains either 1 or 2 percent milk fat, doesn't trim as much fat from your diet as you may think.

Keep in mind that water makes up most of the weight of milk. So once water is eliminated from the calculations, 2 percent milk contains 20 percent fat by weight. What's more, 2 percent milk gets 35 percent of its calories from fat.

Here's one more calculation that may help you make the switch to fat-free. If you drink two glasses of 1 percent milk every day for a year, you're swallowing 4 pounds of fat. Drinking the same amount of fat-free milk, on the other hand, provides less than one-tenth of a pound of fat.

One cup of fat-free milk contains only 0.4 gram of fat, 4 milligrams of cholesterol, and 85 calories. And it has all of the nutrients of whole milk, so you won't lose out on the calcium you need to maintain healthy bones.

CHAPTER FIVE

Supplementing Your Efforts

Gulping down supplements of any kind can't compensate for a high-fat, artery-clogging diet, but research has found that increasing levels of certain vitamins and minerals in food or supplement form can provide cholesterol-lowering benefits and guard against heart disease.

In this chapter, we'll give you the lowdown on some tried-and-true nutrients that are worth considering, as well as some that are only now emerging in research.

ANTIOXIDANTS

Low in fat, high in fiber, and cholesterol-free, fruits and veggies are crucial components of a heart-healthy diet. But there may be another reason to load up on produce. There's evidence that the antioxidant nutrients—vitamins C and E and beta-carotene, which converts to vitamin A in the body—may protect against high blood cholesterol levels. These "supernutrients," which are abundant in fresh fruits and vegetables, may even help prevent heart disease.

Experts believe that antioxidants help thwart a number of chronic illnesses, including heart disease, by foiling the activity of free radicals. The cellular damage caused by these harmful chemical compounds, which are produced both inside and outside the body, can eventually lead to disease. Antioxidant nutrients may help stem this cellular damage.

Furthermore, antioxidants may boost "good" HDL cholesterol and help artery-clogging LDL cholesterol resist oxidation, a chemical process that researchers believe increases the likelihood that LDL cholesterol will collect in the arteries.

Numerous studies associate a high intake of antioxidant nutrients with a lower risk of coronary heart disease and improvement in cholesterol. Many of those studies have found that these benefits occur with doses that are higher than the Daily Values (DVs) for the nutrients. The DV for vitamin C is 60 milligrams; for vitamin E, it's 30 IU. While there is no DV for beta-carotene, some experts recommend consuming just 5 to 6 milligrams daily from foods.

The Antioxidant-Cholesterol Link

"LDL is the major cholesterol-carrying molecule in the bloodstream," says Thomas Bersot, M.D., associate professor of medicine at the University of California, San Francisco. Oxidized LDL is more likely to be trapped by macrophages, a type of cell in the walls of the arteries. When LDL starts to collect inside the macrophages, it sets up a chemical chain reaction that can accelerate oxidation and other artery-clogging processes.

"The accumulation of LDL in the macrophages initiates the entire cascade of events in atherosclerosis," says Dr. Bersot. "If you can prevent LDL from oxidizing, you may reduce the risk of developing hardening of the arteries."

A number of studies have demonstrated an association between a higher intake of antioxidant supplements—particularly vitamins C and E—and a lower risk of heart disease.

Researchers in the Health Professionals' Study, conducted at Harvard Medical School and the Harvard School of Public Health, followed 40,000 healthy male health-care workers for 4 years, tracking how many developed heart disease during that time. They found that the men who consumed the most vitamin E had a lower risk of heart disease. Men who took 100 IU or more of vitamin E daily for at least 2 years cut their risk of heart disease by 37 percent, compared with men who did not take any supplements.

A parallel Harvard study tracked more than 87,000 healthy female nurses for 8 years. Women who consumed the most vitamin E were found to have a 34 percent lower risk of developing heart disease compared with women who consumed the least vitamin E. Women who had taken vitamin E supplements for at least 2 years were 41 percent less likely to develop coronary disease than those who hadn't taken supplements.

At the University of California, Los Angeles, researchers found that men who consumed the most vitamin C had a 45 percent reduction in risk of dying of heart disease; women had a 25 percent reduction in risk. The researchers used data from the first National Health and Nutrition Examination Survey, which included information about the vitamin intakes of more than 11,000 people.

These studies did not specifically explore the relationship between blood cholesterol levels and antioxidants, but other research has examined the possibility that antioxidants may help raise HDL cholesterol and interfere with the oxidation of LDL.

"Several studies have shown that if you progress from consuming a relatively low amount of vitamin C—below 60 milligrams a day—up to 200 to 300 milligrams a day, you'll experience a dose-related increase in HDL cholesterol," says Jeffrey Blumberg, Ph.D., chief of the Antioxidant Research Laboratory at the Jean Mayer USDA Human Nutrition Research Center on Aging at Tufts University in Boston. "This may account for some of the benefits of vitamin C in heart disease."

Researchers at the University of California, San Diego, conducted a two-part study to determine the effects of vitamin E and beta-carotene—used individually, in combination, and together with vitamin C—on the oxidation of LDL. In the first phase, eight people consumed 60 milligrams of beta-carotene per day for 3 months. Then, for another 3 months, they added 1,600 IU of vitamin E a day to the beta-carotene. Finally, for another 3 months, the participants added 2,000 milligrams of vitamin C to the vitamin E and beta-carotene.

In the second phase of the study, the participants consumed only vitamin E supplements (1,600 IU a day) for 5 months. Researchers concluded that long-term use of vitamin E in high doses hindered the oxidation of LDL by 30 to 50 percent. Beta-carotene did not seem to affect LDL's resistance to oxidation.

The Great Debate: Food or Supplements?

Some researchers, including Dr. Blumberg, believe that the DVs—set at levels designed to prevent nutritional deficiencies—are too low to help fight disease. "Going by only the nutritional deficiency criteria, the DVs are absolutely correct," he says. "But if you ask, 'How much vitamin C do I need to reduce my risk of heart disease, cancer, or cataracts?' you'd get a much different answer than the DVs."

What's more, some people may find it difficult to even reach the DVs. In fact, a government survey found that just 9 percent of Americans eat the recommended minimum of five servings of fruits and vegetables a day. And it's difficult to consume potentially therapeutic amounts of some antioxidants through diet alone, say experts.

An important part of the answer, according to Dr. Blumberg, is antioxidant supplements. He recommends consuming between 250 and 1,000 milligrams of vitamin C and between 100 and 400 IU of vitamin E in supplement form. These doses are safe, he says. Since taking large amounts of vitamin C has been reported to cause diarrhea, however, and extremely high doses of vitamin E may cause headaches and diarrhea, be sure to check with your doctor before taking antioxidant supplements.

Because supplements can't compensate for bad dietary habits, it's crucial to follow a healthy diet rich in fruits, vegetables, whole grains, low-fat or fat-free dairy products, and small amounts of lean meat, poultry, and fish. "Rather than relying on supplements, eat foods rich in antioxidants," says Dr. Bersot. "They'll provide antioxidant vitamins as well as other nutritional substances that may be beneficial."

CALCIUM

"Drink your milk! It's good for growing bones."

As a kid, you probably heard this maternal refrain hundreds of times. And Mom was right: Milk—or rather the calcium in milk—does help build strong bones and serve as the first line of defense against osteoporosis.

But along with fracture-proofing your bones, calcium might help protect your ticker by playing a role in lowering blood cholesterol. While the jury is still out on this theory, the evidence is accumulating. Read on.

How Calcium Licks LDL

Heart disease experts have suspected since the 1950s that calcium might lower cholesterol. But most of their studies, while promising, have yielded less-than-sensational results. That's because most of the early research focused on the effects of calcium on total cholesterol. More recent studies have analyzed calcium's effects on the separate components of total cholesterol, LDL (the "bad" kind) and HDL (the "good" kind), which experts consider more sensitive measures of heart disease risk. And the news is encouraging.

Researchers at the University of Texas Southwestern Medical Center at Dallas, led by Margo Denke, M.D., associate professor of medicine in the Center for Human Nutrition, put 13 men with moderately high cholesterol on either a high-calcium diet (2,200 milligrams of calcium per day) or a low-calcium diet (410 milligrams of calcium per day) for 10 weeks. For the next 10 weeks, the men resumed their regular diets. During the study's final 10 weeks, the men who first consumed the high-calcium diet followed the low-calcium plan, and vice versa.

The researchers found that the men's total cholesterol fell an average of 6 percent on the high-calcium diet. Even more significant, their LDL cholesterol dropped an average of 11 percent. Since experts generally agree that every 1 percent decrease in LDL cholesterol results in a 2 percent decrease in heart disease risk, the participants' risk dropped more than 20 percent.

In another study, researchers at the Hennepin County Medical Center in Minneapolis had 56 men and women with mildly to moderately high cholesterol follow a low-fat diet and consume 1,200 milligrams of calcium a day. These folks' LDL cholesterol dropped 4.4 percent, which theoretically decreased their heart disease risk by nearly 10 percent. What's more, their HDL cholesterol increased 4.1 percent.

How might calcium reduce cholesterol? According to the University of Texas study, calcium may both block the absorption of saturated fat and bind with cholesterol-containing bile acids in the digestive system. The body then expels these acids with waste, giving excess cholesterol the boot, too.

Fat-Free Ways to Bone Up Your Diet

Whether the link between increased calcium consumption and lower blood cholesterol will be borne out by further study remains to be seen. Still, "there are many good reasons to increase your calcium intake," says Robert Heaney, M.D., professor of medicine at Creighton University School of Medicine in Omaha, Nebraska, and an expert on calcium.

The most crucial reason? Many people simply don't get enough of this vital mineral. The optimum intake is 1,000 milligrams a day for women age 25 to 50, menopausal women age 51 to 65 who take estrogen, and men age 25 to 65. That amount jumps to 1,500 milligrams a day for menopausal women who don't take estrogen and for all men and women over age 65. Yet it's estimated that 50 percent of women over age 35 consume less than 500 milligrams of calcium a day—far less than they need.

Fortunately, it's easy to fortify your heart and bones with calcium by eating more low-fat or fat-free yogurt, milk, and cheese. Other good sources of the mineral include sardines and canned salmon, calcium-fortified orange juice, and green vegetables like bok choy and kale.

If you suspect that you're not getting enough calcium through your diet, you might consider taking calcium supplements, available in drugstores and health food stores, Dr. Heaney says.

Supplements are not a substitute for a low-fat diet or cholesterol-lowering drugs, if your doctor has prescribed them, says Dr. Denke. But "if you're eating a low-fat, low-saturated-fat, low-cholesterol diet, some additional calcium may be helpful," she says.

Choosing a Calcium Supplement

Dr. Heaney recommends the following guidelines to make sure you get an effective and safe amount of daily supplemental calcium.

• Your body can only absorb up to 500 milligrams of calcium at a time, so don't take a larger amount than that at once.

• Take calcium carbonate—the most common type of calcium supplement—with meals to ensure good absorption. Chewable supplements disintegrate best. Avoid "natural source" calcium carbonate supplements made from bonemeal, dolomite, or oyster shell. Some studies indicate that these products may contain unhealthy amounts of lead.

• Limit your intake of fatty foods, caffeine, alcohol, and tobacco products. All can hinder calcium absorption.

• Don't take calcium supplements with high-fiber wheat bran cereals: These cereals can reduce calcium absorption by 25 percent.

• Make sure to get the Daily Value of vitamin D (400 IU). It's essential for calcium absorption. You can get vitamin D in foods like fat-free milk and some breads and cereals, but consider taking a daily multivitamin/mineral supplement that meets 100 percent of your daily vitamin D requirement.

• Try to avoid calcium supplements that contain aluminum. This chemical can deplete the body's supply of phosphate, which it needs to absorb calcium, Dr. Heaney says.

• Drink lots of water to help avoid constipation, a possible side effect of calcium supplements.

• If you have kidney stones, it's a good idea to check with your doctor before taking calcium supplements. Research indicates, however, that calcium does not heighten the risk of kidney stones, and it may protect against the absorption of oxalic acid, the principal risk factor in the formation of kidney stones.

CHROMIUM

Some of the most intriguing research in the nutritional fight against high cholesterol has to do with a trace mineral whose name reminds most people of the shiny stuff on the bumpers of cars: chromium.

Some studies indicate that chromium, which helps control the way your body uses sugar and fat, may boost the body's stores of "good" HDL cholesterol. "When people who follow a normal diet—which tends to be marginally chromium-deficient—consume more chromium, their cholesterol and triglyceride levels benefit," says Richard A. Anderson, Ph.D., lead scientist at the USDA Human Nutrition Research Center in Beltsville, Maryland, and a leading expert on chromium.

What's more, chromium may help people with glucose intolerance avoid developing type 2 diabetes. Having diabetes increases the risk of developing heart disease.

The Cholesterol Connection

Researchers at Oklahoma State University in Stillwater had 21 people age 60 and over take 150 micrograms of chromium every day for 3 months. Another 21 people took an inactive placebo.

Chromium takers with normal cholesterol exhibited no change in their cholesterol levels. But chromium takers with high cholesterol saw their total cholesterol go down 12 percent and their "bad" LDL cholesterol plummet 14 percent. Just as important, their levels of HDL cholesterol didn't change.

In a second study conducted at Oklahoma State University, 24 people age 55 and over took one of three supplements: chromium (210 micrograms), copper, or zinc. After 2 months, the total cholesterol of the folks taking the chromium fell 12 points, from 217 to 205 milligrams per deciliter (mg/dl) of blood. When they stopped taking the chromium, their total cholesterol crept up again. Copper and zinc had no effect on cholesterol levels.

Getting Enough Chromium

The Daily Value for chromium is 120 micrograms. The average American man consumes 33 micrograms of the mineral a day, and the average woman gets 25 micrograms. "We collected data on 32 people over 7 consecutive days, and not one of them averaged even 50 micrograms of chromium over that one-week period," says Dr. Anderson.

Turkey, grape juice, broccoli, unpeeled apples, green beans, and whole wheat products are good sources of chromium. So, apparently, are some breakfast cereals. "*Total* breakfast cereal is very high in chromium," says Dr. Anderson. "One serving contains nearly 27 micrograms of chromium, which is probably as much as you'll get from everything else you eat all day."

But you need to watch the rest of your diet, too, Dr. Anderson says—especially if you have a sweet tooth. Consuming too many highly processed, sugary foods can rob the body of chromium, which is excreted through the urine. "Eating lots of simple sugars may also increase your need for chromium supplements because you're consuming fewer chromium-rich foods. So you need to pay attention to your overall diet as well as to the amount of chromium you're getting," he says.

Dr. Anderson recommends taking a multivitamin/mineral supplement containing 50 to 200 micrograms of chromium. "One leading brand contains 100 micrograms of chromium," he says. "That extra 100 micrograms a day can serve as an insurance policy should there be a deficiency in your diet."

If you have diabetes, you may need even more chromium, says Dr. Anderson—400 to 600 micrograms a day. Is consuming this amount of chromium safe? Yes, he says. "We've been studying chromium for decades, and we've never documented a single case of a negative effect," he says. Still, it's a good idea to check with your doctor before taking more than a 200-microgram supplement per day.

ARGININE

You probably "take" this possible cholesterol fighter right now without even knowing it. It's arginine, an amino acid found in chicken and all other meats as well as in nuts. The average person eats about 5 grams of it daily.

Your body transforms arginine into a natural substance called nitric oxide, the most potent blood vessel relaxer known. Preliminary research suggests that an extra 6 to 9 milligrams of arginine a day, which may improve coronary bloodflow, can help lower cholesterol levels. How? By acting as an antioxidant and also by keeping blood vessels elastic so that bloodflow is improved and cholesterol deposits are reduced.

Promising, But Not a Sure Thing

The connection between arginine and heart health has not been conclusively shown, however. Robert Eckel, M.D., professor of medicine at the University of Colorado Center for Human Nutrition in Denver and a former chairman of the nutrition committee for the American Heart Association, calls the evidence for arginine a work in progress.

Nevertheless, researcher John Cooke, M.D., associate professor of medicine and director of the vascular section at Stanford University, argues in favor of arginine for certain people.

According to Dr. Cooke, you may want to think about arginine if you're an exerciser with heart or artery disease, since the amino acid may help with bloodflow problems. If this is your situation, it's definitely best to check with your doctor before starting any exercise program or using this supplement. For people with impaired bloodflow to the heart or legs, Dr. Cooke says that those with high cholesterol are most likely to benefit from arginine; people with diabetes and high blood pressure are less likely to respond to it.

Dr. Cooke helped develop HeartBars, which are one of the two sources of arginine other than food. Marketed as a dietary therapy for people with cardiovascular disease, each bar has 180 calories. Eating two a day supplies more than 6 milligrams of arginine as well as other heart-healthy nutrients such as niacin and soy protein.

Arginine is also available in capsules. While they are convenient and easy to swallow, you'd have to take 6 to 18 capsules a day to get the same amount of arginine as in a HeartBar.

Whether you're using HeartBars or capsules, experts say it's a good idea to take your arginine as two or three equal doses taken at different times of the day to maintain even levels in your blood.

PHYTOSTEROLS

Refined from vegetable oils or pine trees, phytosterols play musical chairs with the cholesterol in your intestine, vying for sites in fat-absorbing structures called micelles. If sterols get there first, then cholesterol is left "without a chair" and is flushed out.

Studies done in the 1950s and 1960s showed that phytosterol supplements could lower cholesterol without side effects. Though current products haven't been tested directly, there's every reason to believe that they are just as effective as the popular cholesterol-lowering margarines Benecol and Take Control, which contain phytosterols, says David Kritchevsky, Ph.D., an expert on phytosterols at the Wistar Institute in Philadelphia.

Studies show that 1.5 to 3.3 grams (1,500 to 3,300 milligrams) of phytosterols a day is the most effective dosage. Divide the total dose among all your meals.

Phytosterol products on the market include Kholesterol Blocker with 400 milligrams phytosterols, Source Naturals Phytosterol Complex with 660 milligrams phytosterols, and Natrol Beta-Sitosterol with 300 milligrams phytosterols.

Phytosterols and other cholesterol blockers may lower levels of fat-soluble nutrients such as beta-carotene. So be sure to eat nine or more servings of fruits and vegetables daily to compensate.

SAPONINS

Naturally found in several plants, saponins occur in especially large amounts in alfalfa, soybeans, chickpeas, and yuccaplant. Your body can't absorb saponins, so when they encounter cholesterol in the intestinal tract, they latch onto it and carry it with them when they exit.

Unpublished studies done in Europe show significant reductions in harmful triglycerides, LDL cholesterol, and VLDL cholesterol, and increases in the "good" HDLs. Another study found that monkeys given alfalfa saponins actually experienced a reversal of the artery-clogging process and a 50 percent drop in blood cholesterol levels.

Little is known about standardization, dosage, or effectiveness of these supplements. One such product is Cholestaid, which contains concentrated saponins extracted from alfalfa.

According to Lisa Colodny, Pharm.D., clinical coordinator for pharmacy services at Broward General Medical Center in Fort Lauderdale, Florida, if you try saponin supplements, don't take them instead of your prescription drugs. You'll get the most benefit if you take them together. But check with your doctor first.

FISH OIL CAPSULES

Can you attack high cholesterol by simply swallowing fish oil supplements?

Maybe, maybe not. A few studies suggest that fish oil supplements, which contain beneficial omega-3 fatty acids extracted from fatty fish, may have some health benefits. One study, which examined data on 2,030 men under age 70 who had had heart attacks, found that men who ate salmon, trout, mackerel, or sardines at least twice a week or took three 500-milligram fish oil capsules a day saw their chances of dying during the 2-year study period fall 29 percent.

But some experts say that more studies are needed to prove a relationship between fish oil and lower rates of cardiovascular disease. "There may be instances in which people with very high triglyceride levels can benefit from fish oil capsules," says Wahida Karmally, R.D., director of nutrition at the Irving Center for Clinical Research at Columbia-Presbyterian Medical Center in New York City and a member of the American Heart Association's nutrition committee. "But these capsules have not been shown to lower LDL cholesterol."

Moreover, researchers at Tufts University in Medford, Massachusetts, analyzed popular brands of fish oil supplements and found that they didn't contain sufficient amounts of vitamin E, which is added to help keep the omega-3s in the capsules from breaking down.

So what's the bottom line? "The best way to consume any nutrient is to consume it in food," says Susan Kleiner, R.D., Ph.D., a nutritionist in Seattle and author of *The High-Performance Cookbook*. "Our bodies absorb nutrients most efficiently through food."

If you do choose to take omega-3 supplements, however, consult your doctor first, Dr. Kleiner says. Some research shows that large doses of fish oil may thin the blood and may raise the risk of excessive bleeding or stroke. For these reasons, the American Heart Association advises people to take fish oil supplements only under a doctor's supervision.

CHAPTER SIX

The Power of Plants

Like foods, some herbal remedies contain chemicals that may have cholesterol-lowering properties. The following herbs might be worth considering as you plan your options for getting your cholesterol in check.

ARTICHOKE EXTRACT

Artichokes are a springtime staple, but research now shows that they can have year-round benefits.

German researchers gave 143 men and women who had elevated levels of total cholesterol (more than 280 milligrams per deciliter, or mg/dl) either 1,800 milligrams of dried artichoke extract or an inactive placebo every day for 6 weeks. By the study's end, those who took the extract lowered their cholesterol levels by an average of 18 percent. The placebo group's cholesterol dropped by about 8 percent. In addition, the researchers found that levels of "bad" LDL cholesterol fell more than 20 percent in the people who took the extract and that the ratio of protective HDL to LDL also improved.

Even better, there were no drug-related side effects reported during the study.

Artichokes contain a compound called cynarin, which increases production of bile by the liver. Studies also show that the extract boosts the flow of bile from the gallbladder. Bile plays a key role in the excretion of excess cholesterol from the body.

Artichoke supplements can be found at most health food stores. If you're using dried artichoke leaf, take 2 grams three times a day; if using artichoke leaf 2:1 tincture, take 1 milliliter (20 drops) three times a day; if using a standardized artichoke extract, follow the instructions on the label.

GARLIC EXTRACT

As we learned in chapter 4, garlic can be a powerful—albeit powerful-smelling—ally against cholesterol.

If, however, you just can't tolerate the herb's aroma, garlic extract may be helpful, too.

Researchers at Tulane University School of Medicine in New Orleans gave 42 men and women with elevated cholesterol either 900 milligrams of garlic extract (divided among three capsules) or a placebo every day. After 12 weeks, the total cholesterol of the folks taking the garlic extract fell 6 percent, from 262 to 247 mg/dl, and their LDL cholesterol plunged 11 percent, from 188 to 168 mg/dl. By contrast, the total and LDL cholesterol of those consuming the placebo fell only 1 and 3 percent, respectively.

Garlic supplements are available in health food stores and most drugstores. One such supplement, Kwai pow-ier tablets, contains the equivalent of 2.7 grams of fresh garlic—or nearly one clove—in each 900-milligram dose.

GUGGUL

This supplement has gotten a lot of attention lately for its heart-healthy benefits. Guggul is actually the hardened sap, or resin, of an Indian desert tree. This Ayurvedic remedy has been around for many years and has been used by Indian physicians to treat immune system disorders such as rheumatoid arthritis. More recently it has been shown to reduce levels of cholesterol and other blood fats.

How does it work? Some studies, most conducted in India, have identified several active components of guggul. Two of these, gugulipid and guggulsterone, lowered blood fats (cholesterol and triglycerides) significantly in small animals and in people. The theory is that guggul encourages the liver to specifically burn fat and cholesterol.

One study in India showed that 80 percent of people who used guggul extract had a 30 percent drop in levels of cholesterol and other blood fats. Some nutrition experts in the United States remain skeptical about the quality of that research, however.

Although guggul was also a traditional cure for obesity, it's not a magic bullet. It may *help* reduce body fat and cholesterol, but only in tandem with a sensible diet and exercise.

Guggul appears to be quite safe, although some people report occasional stomach upset. People with overactive thyroids should avoid guggul, and it should never be used by pregnant women because it can stimulate uterine contractions.

If your doctor gives guggul the go-ahead, look for a product marked "standardized" to gugulipids and take 500 milligrams twice a day.

HAWTHORN

Experts believe hawthorn is the best herb overall for heart health. Some research suggests that it lowers cholesterol, too.

The hawthorn berry compounds suspected of benefiting cholesterol—beta-sitosterol, catechin, chromium, fiber, linoleic acid, magnesium, pectin, and rutin—may also contribute to the herb's blood pressure–lowering effects.

Look for a product made with hawthorn extract that's standardized to contain 1.8 percent of a compound called vitexin. Take 100 milligrams three times a day.

Anyone with a heart condition should not take hawthorn regularly for more than a few weeks without medical supervision. Your doctor may need to adjust your dosage of other medications. Likewise, if you have low blood pressure caused by heart valve problems, do not use hawthorn without medical supervision.

RED YEAST RICE EXTRACT

Cultivated on rice, red yeast contains natural substances that are chemically similar to the active ingredients in statin drugs that are widely prescribed for high cholesterol. It appears that these substances, technically known as HMG-CoA reductase inhibitors, stimulate the formation of good HDL cholesterol and reduce the production of bad LDL cholesterol.

Clinical trials showed that daily consumption of four 600-milligram capsules of a standardized red yeast product called Cholestin produced significant reductions in blood levels of both cholesterol and triglycerides (another blood fat implicated in heart disease).

The first U.S. study of Cholestin involved 83 people with high cholesterol. The 42 who took Cholestin for 12 weeks lowered their total cholesterol by an average of 16 percent. From a total cholesterol level of 250, that's a drop of 40 points.

Cholestin also contains unsaturated fatty acids that appear to lower triglycerides, and at the same time, it appears to increase levels of beneficial HDL cholesterol.

In 1998, the FDA banned over-the-counter sales of Cholestin because it deemed that its active ingredients were too closely related to lovastatin, a prescription drug sold as Mevacor, and therefore infringed on patents for that drug. Pharmanex, the maker of Cholestin, has since been ordered to discontinue sale of the product.

Currently, generic red yeast rice extracts (sometimes called Chinese red yeast) are available. These products may be neither safe nor effective, however. Specific claims for the cholesterol-lowering benefits of generic red yeast rice extract are often based on research on Cholestin, not on the generic supplements.

"A recent analysis found that many of these products, which aren't as well-studied as Cholestin, contain lower levels of the cholesterol-lowering compounds," says Andrew T. Weil, M.D., clinical professor of medicine and director of the program in integrative medicine at the University of Arizona in Tucson and editor of *Dr. An-*

drew Weil's Self-Healing newsletter. "Plus, some are contaminated with citrinin, a toxin that causes kidney damage in animals."

Cholestin is less likely to cause liver dysfunction than prescription statin drugs. In the event that the product becomes available again, anyone with a history of liver disease should use it with caution. For now, generic red yeast extract should also be used cautiously, if at all. It isn't recommended for use by people who are under age 20 or by women who are pregnant or nursing.

With so many other safe and effective ways to lower your cholesterol, as outlined throughout this book, generic red yeast rice extract may not be worth the risk at this time.

PART III

Managing Cholesterol for a Lifetime

As you've already learned, the first treatments that doctors frequently recommend to tame high cholesterol are actions that are totally under your control—fixing your diet, getting more exercise, and losing weight.

In theory, that sounds great. But in real life, it's not always so easy.

In this section, you'll learn exactly how to eat smarter, how to make exercise more appealing, and how to drop those stubborn pounds. You'll also get the facts on two more topics of importance to heart-friendly, low-cholesterol living: reducing your stress and cutting down on unhealthy habits.

CHAPTER SEVEN

Eat a Healthy Diet

MEAL FREQUENCY

It sounds too good to be true: being able to eat all day long and lower your blood cholesterol in the process. But there's some evidence that "grazing"—eating many small meals or snacks rather than the more customary three squares a day—can help shave a few points off your cholesterol level.

But don't confuse eating more often with consuming more calories, experts say. Grazing on hot fudge sundaes and hero sandwiches will benefit neither your cholesterol level nor your shape. "We're recommending not that people eat more calories but that they divide their daily caloric intakes into smaller meals," says Elizabeth Barrett-Connor, M.D., professor and chairperson of the department of family medicine at the University of California, San Diego.

The good news is that studies indicate that the cholesterol-lowering benefits of eating smaller, more frequent meals seem to take effect without changing your overall diet. How's that for a dream come true?

It Pays to Graze

Grazing may be the natural way to eat, Dr. Barrett-Connor says. "We evolved from people who ate frequent, small meals when they could," she says. "Occasionally, they would get a big kill and gorge. But Americans gorge nearly every night—and that's very unhealthy."

The body manages smaller meals more efficiently, explains Sharon Edelstein, a research scientist at George Washington University in Washington, D.C. "Humans were meant to be grazers, and that's the way our bodies perform best," she says. "If you pound your body with a lot of food once or twice a day, you may be giving it too much to deal with. If you put food into your body more slowly, you'll process it more efficiently."

Dr. Barrett-Connor agrees. "Eating more meals consisting of less food is more physiologically efficient," she says. "If you throw large amounts of fat and calories at the body all at once, it won't be able to manage them as well. It's more than the body can metabolize." So fueling up only once or twice a day may make it easier for dietary fat to collect in the coronary arteries, leading to elevated cholesterol levels.

If you'd like more evidence that eating smaller portions may affect heart health, look at countries that have lower incidences of cardiovascular disease than the United States, such as Japan and China, suggests Marla Mendelson, M.D., assistant professor of medicine at Northwestern University Medical School in Chicago. "The people in these countries eat smaller portions," she says. "This may aid the digestive process, so you're not completely overwhelming the mechanism in the liver with too much food and asking the liver to process it." Overloading the liver may eventually cause free-floating fat and cholesterol to be deposited in the arteries, she says.

Four (or More) Meals Are Better Than One

Researchers found that when laboratory animals ate large, infrequent meals rather than small, frequent ones, their blood cholesterol increased. Multiple feedings resulted in reduced heart disease risk factors—and longer lives, Dr. Barrett-Connor says.

Studies conducted on humans appear to bear out the conclusions of the animal research. Edelstein and Dr. Barrett-Connor, along with other colleagues, studied the diets of more than 2,000 people. They found that the total cholesterol of people who ate four or more meals a day was almost 9 points lower than those who reported eating one or two meals a day, says Dr. Barrett-Connor. Also, the frequent eaters' "bad" LDL cholesterol averaged six points lower than that of the infrequent eaters, she says.

Researchers in New Zealand had 19 healthy men and women with normal blood cholesterol levels consume their usual low-fat diets—with one difference: These folks alternated between eating three meals a day and eating nine meals a day. They spent 2 weeks on each diet. When the participants followed the nine-meal plan, their total cholesterol fell 6.5 percent, and their LDL cholesterol dropped 8.1 percent.

Thinking of joining the graze craze? These tips can help.

• People who eat breakfast generally eat more meals a day than people who don't, Dr. Barrett-Connor says. Breakfast-eaters also are more likely to snack throughout the day than people who diet all day long and eat gigantic dinners. In fact, people who skip breakfast to "save" calories end up spending them—with interest—in the long run. "Their bodies store up fat for the famine they think is coming," she says.

• Many weight-control experts recommend that people eat a small snack between meals and another snack before bedtime, Dr. Barrett-Connor says. Snacking between meals provides the body with the same amount of calories but is more physiologically efficient. "Avoid foods high in fat or sugar—they have no nutritional value," she advises. "Fruits and vegetables are great choices."

FOOD AND NUTRITION FACTORS

While snacking throughout the day instead of eating large meals is helpful, you obviously can't snack on just anything. Certain foods—namely eggs, meat, margarine, and cheese—are often cited for their role in raising cholesterol, so you'll want to watch them carefully. If, however, you eat only moderate portions of these foods, they can certainly continue to be a part of your diet. Let's take a closer look at each one.

Eggs

Can't remember the last time you ate a three-egg omelette? You're not alone. Many people have cut down on eggs—or even given them up entirely—as part of their efforts to lower their cholesterol.

Eggs definitely have their good points, however. One large egg is brimming with vitamins E and B_{12}, folate, riboflavin, phosphorus, and iron, with less than 2 grams of saturated fat. They pack plenty of protein, too. "Eggs are the best-quality, least expensive protein we can eat," says Wanda Howell, R.D., Ph.D., assistant professor of nutritional sciences at the University of Arizona in Tucson.

So why can't we enjoy eggs as often as we wish? Because most of the protein in the egg is in the white; all of the cholesterol is in the yolk, explains Dean Ornish, M.D., president and director of the Preventive Medicine Research Institute in Sausalito, California, and author of *Dr. Dean Ornish's Program for Reversing Heart Disease*. The yolk of one average egg contains

213 milligrams of dietary cholesterol—more than two-thirds of the daily limit of 300 milligrams recommended by the American Heart Association (AHA).

The AHA says that healthy adults can eat up to four whole eggs per week but advises people with elevated cholesterol to limit themselves to one whole egg a week. "Because eggs—or more specifically, egg yolks—are a concentrated source of dietary cholesterol, you shouldn't overdo them," says Chicago dietitian Alicia Moag-Stahlberg, R.D., a spokesperson for the American Dietetic Association.

In one study, 25 people were asked to eat 12 eggs a week for 6 weeks. In 23 of the participants, cholesterol levels stayed the same. In the other 2, LDL cholesterol rose by 25 percent. That translates into a 50 percent increase in the estimated risk of a heart attack.

Evidently, eating eggs doesn't necessarily raise blood levels of cholesterol in everyone. The term *responders* was used by the researchers to describe the people whose LDL increased. There's no way to know if you'll be a responder, so study author Nancy Lewis, R.D., Ph.D., a nutritionist at the University of Nebraska in Lincoln, recommends that you have your cholesterol checked a month or so after adding eggs to your diet. If your numbers have spiked upward, switch back to egg substitutes. These products consist primarily of egg whites, with other ingredients—including fat-free milk, food coloring, vegetable oil, and vitamins—added to mimic the taste and texture of real eggs and to boost nutritional value.

Here's how to use egg substitutes, egg whites—and the occasional whole egg—as part of an overall low-fat, low-cholesterol diet.

• It's possible for you to create an appetizing breakfast without using whole eggs. "You don't have to sacrifice flavor," says Evelyn Tribole, R.D., a dietitian in Beverly Hills, California, and author of *Healthy Homestyle Cooking*. "Try making French toast with egg whites and fat-free milk. Or make egg-white omelettes stuffed with bell peppers, mushrooms, and onions. Chopped green chile peppers work well, too." But don't sauté all of those vegetables in butter. Use a cooking spray instead.

• If you have tried egg substitute in the past but didn't care for it, you may want to try it again, Tribole says. "Some of the newer egg substitutes taste much more like real eggs," she says. And the more brands you try, the more likely it is that you'll find one you like. There's one advantage of using egg substitute over egg whites, says Tribole: It's yellow, so it looks like the real thing. "If you like scrambled eggs and you're really into eye appeal, use egg substitute," she says. And with more and more restaurants offering omelettes and scrambled eggs made with egg substitute, it's not difficult to follow your program away from home.

• If you must have the real thing, "buy small or medium-size eggs, which contain a little less cholesterol than larger eggs," suggests James W. Anderson, M.D., professor of medicine and clinical nutrition at the University of Kentucky College of Medicine in Lexington.

• Don't scramble or fry eggs in bacon grease or butter, as both are full of saturated fat. Instead, prepare them in a nonstick skillet coated with a cooking spray. Or try eating eggs hard-boiled or poached, Dr. Howell suggests.

• As mentioned, one egg accounts for most of the AHA's recommended daily intake of dietary cholesterol. "So if you eat an egg on Sunday, make Monday an egg-free or low-cholesterol day," says Sheah Rarback, R.D., director of nutrition at the Mailman Center at the University of Miami School of Medicine. "Concern yourself not with every meal, or even with every mouthful, but with your diet as a whole."

Meat

If you have elevated cholesterol, you must avoid red meat. Right?

Not necessarily. Despite what you may have heard, experts say that you don't have to forgo steak and burgers entirely to keep tabs on your cholesterol. The key to making red meat part of a low-fat, low-cholesterol diet is to eat smaller portions of leaner cuts, says Susan Kleiner, R.D., Ph.D., a nutritionist in Seattle and author of *The High-Performance Cookbook.*

Red meat is a great source of protein, iron, zinc, and B vitamins. But a little bit of it goes a long way, and experts advise against broiling up a steak too often. "Red meat is high in saturated fat, so you shouldn't overdo it," says Janet Lepke, R.D., a dietitian in Santa Monica, California, and a spokesperson for the American Dietetic Association.

Because cattle are being raised differently and because meat processors are trimming away visible fat, in some cases red meat is lower in fat, cholesterol, and calories than it used to be. In fact, "some of the leaner cuts of red meat contain less fat than skinless chicken thighs," says Tammy Baker, R.D., a nutritionist in Cave Creek, Arizona, and a spokesperson for the American Dietetic Association.

A few studies have beefed up the argument that red

meat can be part of a cholesterol-lowering diet.

In a study at Baylor College of Medicine in Houston, two groups of men with high blood cholesterol levels were placed on a 5-week stabilization diet in which 40 percent of their calories came from fat. These men then switched to one of two low-fat test diets in which they ate either chicken breast or lean beef (choice strip loin steak) for 5 more weeks. The beef contained 8 percent fat, and the chicken, 7 percent fat.

After 5 weeks, both groups' total cholesterol decreased significantly—7.6 percent for the meat-eaters and 10.2 percent for the poultry-eaters. The men's "bad" LDL cholesterol also dropped significantly on both diets, although not to desirable levels. The researchers concluded that lean beef and chicken are interchangeable in a low-fat, low-cholesterol diet.

In an Australian study, researchers placed 10 people on a very low fat diet that contained lean beef with the fat trimmed off. The participants' total cholesterol fell significantly within a week. But when beef fat (in the form of drippings) was added to these folks' diet, their total cholesterol rose. The researchers concluded that it was the beef fat, not the beef itself, that raised blood cholesterol. Further, they wrote, the low-fat diet with lean beef (but without the fat drippings) was just as effective at lowering cholesterol as other low-fat diets that were tested.

To make red meat part of your low-fat, low-cholesterol diet, keep these shopping guidelines and serving suggestions in mind.

- Eat red meat only a couple times a week and keep the servings small, Baker advises. "The suggested serving size is about 3 ounces," she says. "That's a little smaller than the palm of your hand or about the size of a deck of cards." Agrees Dr. Kleiner, "Sixteen-ounce steaks are no longer the way to go."

• Choose the leanest cuts of meat. If you're shopping for pork, select the tenderloin, leg, and shoulder. If you're buying lamb, choose the arm and loin.

• The leanest cuts of beef usually carry the label "USDA select." On average, select beef contains 20 percent less fat than "choice" beef and 40 percent less fat than "prime." Extra-lean ground beef contains just 10 percent fat based on weight.

• You can estimate the fat content of a cut of meat just by looking at it, according to Mary Donkersloot, R.D., a dietitian in Beverly Hills, California, a spokesperson for the California Dietetic Association, and author of *The Fast Food Diet*. "Check to see how much white marbling the meat has," she suggests. The more marbling, the more fat.

• Cut away all visible fat from red meat before you cook it. While trimming the fat won't affect taste much, it will dramatically reduce your intake of fat and calories.

• "If you eat meat, broil it," suggests Gene A. Spiller, D.Sc., Ph.D., director of the Health Research and Studies Center in Los Altos, California, and author of *The Super-pyramid Eating Program*. "Let the fat drip off the meat, but don't let it drain on hot charcoal or a hot burner, which will create undesirable fumes."

• Substitute whole or ground turkey or chicken in recipes that call for beef. Make turkey burgers instead of hamburgers, or meat loaf with ground turkey instead of ground beef. "But the less fatty the meat is, the drier it can get," says Tribole. She suggests adding a medium-size grated apple to a pound of ground turkey. "The apple will give the turkey a nice texture without adding extra fat," she says.

• "Marinate meat in something flavorful," suggests Marilyn Cerino, R.D., nutrition consultant at the Benjamin Franklin Center for Health of Pennsylvania Hospital in Philadelphia. One savory marinade is a blend of fresh orange juice, light soy sauce, olive oil, garlic, and ginger. "You can use this mixture to marinate strips of meat or chicken that you plan to stir-fry," Cerino says. "And if the meat is tough, marinate it overnight."

Margarine

Many men and women who are watching their cholesterol have abandoned butter. Instead, the stuff that about three of every four Americans spread on their morning toast is margarine.

Now, however, we're hearing about significant evidence suggesting that trans fatty acids, a type of fat found in margarine as well as a lot of snacks and baked goods, raise "bad" LDL cholesterol, lower "good" HDL cholesterol, and increase the risk of heart attack.

Thankfully, the news isn't all bad. Much depends on the type of margarine you select. The softer the margarine is (such as tub and liquid forms), the fewer trans fatty acids it contains.

Trans fatty acids are by-products of innovations in food technology. Margarine is made mostly from unsaturated oils, such as corn, canola, and safflower, to name a few. Unsaturated oils are liquid at room temperature. To solidify them, manufacturers pump them up with hydrogen in a chemical process called hydrogenation. So stick margarine is more hydrogenated than a tub of soft margarine.

Hydrogenation also creates trans fatty acids. Ironically, when unsaturated fatty acids are chemically combined with hydrogen, they become more saturated.

Despite this, however, some experts, including the American Heart Association, still say that it's better to opt for margarine over butter. Why? Because butter has more artery-clogging saturated fat, which has been proven to elevate blood cholesterol and raise the risk of heart disease. Butter contains about 7 grams of saturated fat per tablespoon; margarine has only about 2 grams per tablespoon.

"Studies show that while both trans fatty acids and saturated fat increase LDL cholesterol, saturated fat has a greater effect on cholesterol," says Moag-Stahlberg. Further, we consume far more saturated fat. "About 3 percent of our total calories come from trans fatty acids, compared with 12 to 13 percent from saturated fat," she says.

For now, experts say, your best bet is to concentrate on cutting back on saturated fat. If you're still using butter, switching to margarine can be a good start.

With so many varieties of margarine to choose from, picking a truly heart-healthy product can be tricky. These guidelines can help.

- First and foremost, select a margarine that contains no more than 2 grams of saturated fat per tablespoon, advises the AHA. "Choose only margarines that list water as the first ingredient," advises William P. Castelli, M.D., medical director of the Framingham Cardiovascular Institute, a wellness program at Metro West Medical Center in Massachusetts. These products are low in trans fatty acids as well as in saturated fat, he explains. "And avoid margarine that lists partially hydrogenated vegetable oil as the first ingredient," he says. Instead, use products with naturally occurring, unhydrogenated oil such as canola or olive oil when possible.

• Consider switching to a new cholesterol-lowering spread, such as Benecol or Take Control, which are made with plant stanol esters. These ingredients lower cholesterol by blocking its absorption in the body.

• Avoid stick margarine, as it tends to be highly hydrogenated. Opt for soft, tub-style margarine instead, suggests Alice H. Lichtenstein, D.Sc., assistant professor of nutrition at Tufts University in Medford, Massachusetts, and a scientist at the Jean Mayer USDA Human Nutrition Research Center on Aging in Boston.

• Select a brand with the highest percentage of polyunsaturated fat, Dr. Lichtenstein advises. You might opt for products made from safflower, sunflower, corn, or soybean oil.

• Skip the spread altogether. "We've been raised to think that we should smear something on our toast," Dr. Lichtenstein says. "But if we eat tasty bread, we may not need to." Another option: Top your toast with a small amount of jelly or jam, which contains no saturated fat.

Cheese

If you're trying to avoid heart disease, eating too much rich, creamy cheese can raise your blood cholesterol and clog your coronary arteries faster than you can say "double-cheese pizza."

Cheese is little more than a concentrated form of milk.

It takes about 8 pounds of milk to create a single pound of most cheeses. Many full-fat cheeses get 60 percent or more of their calories from fat, and 1 ounce of Cheddar, Swiss, Monterey Jack, or Muenster contains 8 to 10 grams of fat. Just reading a cheese label with those kinds of numbers is enough to make your arteries slam shut!

The good news is that the dairy industry has responded to the public's demands for healthier cheese by introducing some products that get 10 percent or less of their calories from fat and contain 2 grams or less of fat per ounce.

The key to choosing heart-healthy cheese, experts say, is to become a dedicated label reader. Select cheeses with low amounts of total fat and saturated fat and low percentages of calories from fat, advises Rarback.

How low is low enough? "Choose a cheese in which the percentage of fat is lower than the percentage of protein," says Dr. Spiller. A product that is 20 percent fat and 15 percent protein, for example, should stay out of your shopping cart, he says.

Also, when it comes to controlling blood cholesterol, a cheese's fat content is more important than its dietary cholesterol, says Ruth Lowenberg, R.D., a dietitian in New York City. The American Heart Association recommends that adults eat less than 300 milligrams of dietary cholesterol per day. Don't be misled, however: A 1-ounce serving of American cheese contains 26 milligrams of cholesterol but 9 grams of fat—a hefty amount if you're trying to follow a low-fat diet.

These hints can help you make low-fat and fat-free cheeses more palatable.

• Look for low-fat "impostors." Chances are there's a low-fat or fat-free alternative for your favorite type of full-fat cheese, including Cheddar (Healthy Choice Fat-Free, Cracker Barrel Light), mozzarella (Kraft Healthy Favorites, Alpine Lace Low Moisture Part-Skim), Swiss (Light 'n' Lively Singles, Kraft Light Naturals), and American (Weight Watchers Slices, Kraft Free Singles). "Do some taste-testing," Tribole says. "You may find that there's a considerable difference in taste among brands of the same type of cheese."

• Try combining small amounts of a higher-fat cheese with a low-fat or fat-free product. "You might add cubes of low-fat mozzarella to a salad, then sprinkle the salad with blue cheese," Lowenberg suggests. "You'll get a wonderful cheesy flavor without using a large amount of the higher-fat cheese."

• Using condiments can give a fat-free cheese some extra zip. "If you're using a fat-free cheese in a sandwich, you may not be able to get away with adding just lettuce and tomato," Lowenberg says. "Try spreading on some horseradish or chutney, which will enhance the cheese's flavor."

• Love the taste of creamy cheeses such as Brie? Try this mock Brie dish, suggests Sue Chapman, executive chef at Skylonda Fitness Retreat in Woodside, California: Mix one part Brie cheese, four parts fat-free cream cheese, and some rosemary; shape into rounds; and dip in bread crumbs. Then bake.

• The next time you make lasagna, substitute reduced-fat ricotta cheese for the whole-milk product. A half-cup of reduced-fat ricotta contains 9.8 grams of fat, compared with 16.1 grams in the same amount of the whole-milk stuff.

• **Fat-free cheeses don't melt very well.** So don't use these products to top casseroles, advises Tribole. "Fat-free cheese will look like toasted coconut," she says. "I'd use a low-fat cheese instead." Similarly, fat-free mozzarella works better baked into lasagna than on a pizza, she notes. But if you want to use a fat-free cheese in a sauce, "try shredding it very finely," she suggests. "It will melt nicely."

CHAPTER EIGHT

Get Moving

If "surfing" the Internet and "running" through the TV channels with your remote control are your main forms of exercise, you're not alone. Only about 1 in 10 of us is physically active for ½ hour or more a day.

But if you have high cholesterol and you've been sedentary, one of the best things that you can do for your heart is to get moving. Among its many benefits, regular exercise can lower your LDL level, raise your HDL level, and help you maintain a healthy weight. Physical activity can also control other risk factors for heart disease, including high blood pressure.

Getting into the exercise habit can be easier than you think, even if you haven't worked up a sweat in years. What's more, many experts say, ½ hour of exercise a day is all that it takes to improve your cholesterol profile and reduce your risk of developing heart disease, high blood pressure, and diabetes. The simple, inexpensive practice of walking may be your best bet.

Want to exchange 30 minutes of channel flipping a

day for a lifetime of good health? You can. Read on to find out how.

THE DREAM TEAM

According to scientific evidence, exercise helps boost levels of "good" HDL cholesterol, which helps whisk "bad" LDL cholesterol out of the body. "It is thought that exercise's ability to reduce the risk of heart disease comes mostly from its ability to increase HDL cholesterol," says James Rippe, M.D., director of the Center for Clinical and Lifestyle Research at Tufts University School of Medicine in Boston and coauthor of *Dr. James Rippe's Complete Book of Fitness Walking.*

A high HDL level is associated with a decreased risk of heart disease. For every 1-point increase in HDL, risk of heart disease sinks by 2 percent for men and 3 percent for women. So if you're a woman who raises your HDL reading from 45 to 55 milligrams/deciliter (mg/dl), you'll slash your risk of heart disease by about 30 percent!

In one study, doctors in Thailand surveyed 3,615 people for their risk factors for heart disease and for their levels of physical activity. The researchers found that people who exercised regularly were more likely to have lower triglyceride levels and resting heart rates. Additionally, levels of HDL cholesterol were higher in men and women who exercised regularly.

Physical activity appears to trigger a chain of physiological events that increase the efficiency of an enzyme called lipoprotein lipase, says Michael Miller, M.D., director of preventive cardiology at the University of Maryland School of Medicine in Baltimore. This enzyme attacks triglycerides. "As lipoprotein lipase breaks down triglyceride-rich particles, it also produces substances that help make HDL," Dr. Miller says. So people who exercise tend to make more HDL and have lower triglyceride levels.

CYCLE, GOLF ... OR JUST SCRUB THE TUB

Think you have to become a marathon runner to raise your HDL and slash your risk of heart disease? Nope. Again, the magic number is 30 minutes of moderate-intensity exercise a day, say experts convened by the Centers for Disease Control and Prevention and the American College of Sports Medicine. According to these experts, "the scientific evidence clearly demonstrates that regular, moderate-intensity physical activity provides substantial health benefits."

Experts define moderate exercise as the equivalent of walking 2 miles at a brisk pace. Other moderate-intensity activities include cycling for pleasure, playing golf (pulling the cart or carrying clubs), cleaning the house, and mowing the lawn with a power mower.

Even better, you can accumulate this 30-minute minimum in short bursts of activity rather than all at once, experts say. So walking instead of driving short distances or pedaling a stationary bicycle while you watch your favorite sitcom can confer substantial health benefits.

Consult your doctor before you start any exercise program, particularly if you are a woman over age 50 or a man over age 40, are overweight, have diabetes or heart disease, or have ever fainted or experienced chest pains while exercising. And remember to start slowly and listen to your body. "Intense physical activity in people who are not used to it is very dangerous," says William P. Castelli, M.D., medical director of the Framingham Cardiovascular Institute, a wellness program at Metro West Medical Center in Massachusetts.

WALKING: PARTICULARLY GOOD EXERCISE

"Walking is man's best medicine," said the Greek physician Hippocrates. If the good doctor were around today, he'd add that regular constitutionals can benefit *women*, too. In fact, walking is good medicine for virtually everyone, no matter what their age or level of fitness.

Studies have shown that walking can help improve your cholesterol profile as well as lower blood pressure, reduce the risk of heart attack and stroke, and control diabetes. "Walking may be the best medicine, because you can do it forever," Dr. Castelli says.

What's more, you don't need to own a closetful of expensive gear to reap the benefits of this simple yet effective exercise, experts say. "Walking is convenient and easy to do, and requires no special equipment," says Darlene A. Sedlock, Ph.D., associate professor of kinesiology at Purdue University in West Lafayette, Indiana. "You can just step out your door and go."

Investigators at the Institute for Aerobics Research in Dallas gave treadmill tests to more than 13,000 people and followed their fitness levels for 8 years. They discovered that folks who walked for ½ hour a day had reduced levels of premature death nearly as impressive as those of people who ran 30 to 40 miles a week.

You don't have to power-walk to prevent heart disease and promote health. Walking briskly for 2 miles every day, or nearly every day, is a great way to accumulate the expert-recommended ½ hour of physical activity a day. What's more, speed doesn't determine effectiveness.

Researchers at the Institute for Aerobics Research had 59 women walk 3 miles a day, 5 days a week, for 6 months. But their speeds varied. The first group of women walked a mile in 12 minutes. The second group walked a mile in 15 minutes. And the third group took 20 minutes to walk a mile. The fastest group of women had more impressive improvements in their overall fitness than the slowest group. But the HDL levels of all three groups jumped an average of 6 percent.

The bottom line? Speed and distance are less important than consistency, experts say. "It's more important to walk at a comfortable pace on a regular basis," says Dan Rench, R.N., program director for cardiovascular rehabilitation at the Indiana Heart Institute at St. Vincent Hospital in Indianapolis. "If walking is fun, you'll probably stick with it."

"You should be able to carry on a conversation while you walk," adds exercise physiologist Peter Snell, Ph.D., assistant professor of internal medicine at the University of Texas Southwestern Medical Center at Dallas. If you're gasping for breath while you try to talk, slow down.

KNOCK DOWN CHOLESTEROL WITH EXERCISE AND DIET

While exercise has been proven to lower the risk of coronary heart disease, exercise combined with a low-fat diet can pack an even stronger punch.

READY, SET, WALK!
Ready to hit the road? These expert tips can help you keep pace.

• Invest in a good pair of walking shoes. While you don't need hundred-dollar footwear, "you need more than ordinary tennis shoes for walking," says James Rippe, M.D., director of the Center for Clinical and Lifestyle Research at Tufts University School of Medicine in Boston and coauthor of *Dr. James Rippe's Complete Book of Fitness Walking*.

The shoes you choose should be lightweight and padded at the heel and tongue as well as have an absorbent lining. Also, the shoe should bend easily across the ball of your foot and feature an up-tilted sole to enhance your natural walking motion.

• Find a walking buddy, suggests Michael Miller, M.D., director of preventive cardiology at the University of Maryland School of Medicine in Baltimore. Invite a coworker to take a "walk break" instead of a coffee break, then go for a 15-minute stroll. You might even ask your spouse to share your walk before or after work.

• In hot weather, wear loose-fitting, lightweight clothes, Dr. Rippe advises. And try to walk in the early morning or early evening, when the heat is less intense. Drink lots of water before and during your walk.

• In cold weather, dress in light layers that you can easily remove as your body warms up. "And watch your footing—your path could be icy and hazardous," Dr. Miller says. In truly stormy weather, climb up and down the stairs at home. *Caution:* If you have heart disease, diabetes, asthma, or other health conditions, consult your doctor before walking in cold weather.

• Join a local walking club, Dr. Miller suggests. If you can't find one, consider starting your own.

• Forge new paths. Explore the grounds of a nearby botanical garden on foot. Or buy a book of local walking tours and hit the road.

Researchers in Germany had one group of men with chest pain exercise at home for ½ hour a day as well as participate in two 1-hour group exercise sessions per week. The men also followed a low-fat, low-cholesterol diet. Another group of men was encouraged—but not required—to exercise regularly and consume a low-fat diet.

After a year, the LDL cholesterol of the men who both dieted and exercised dropped an average of 8 percent, and their HDL climbed 3 percent. What's more, only 23 percent of the men experienced progression in existing blockages in their coronary arteries. In another 32 percent, the disease process actually regressed. By contrast, the LDL and HDL cholesterol of the men in the control group didn't change, and 48 percent experienced progression of existing arterial blockages.

Researchers at Stanford University School of Medicine, led by Peter Wood, D.Sc., Ph.D., professor emeritus of medicine, had one group of moderately overweight people follow a low-fat, low-cholesterol diet. A second group followed the same diet but also exercised three times a week. After a year, the exercisers raised their HDL levels an average of 13 percent. By contrast, the diet-only group raised their HDL 2 percent.

NINE HEART-HEALTHY FITNESS TIPS

There's no denying the proven benefits of regular exercise, from a healthier heart to a better shape. So don your sweats and get moving! These tips can help make it easier.

Put your workout in writing. You're more likely to stick to an exercise program if you document what you're doing, Dr. Snell says. "Start keeping a workout log," he suggests. "The log will be a record of your accomplishments and will help keep you on track."

Find activities you enjoy. From fencing to inline skating to yoga, there's a wealth of fitness options that you may not have considered. So explore the alternatives. "When you're having fun being physically active, you're much more likely to keep going, week after week and month after month," Dr. Sedlock says.

Go at your own pace. "Don't adhere to the adage 'No pain, no gain,' " Dr. Sedlock says. "Do what you're capable of doing. You'll find that exercise becomes easier and easier."

Schedule a "happy hour" for exercise. "If you commit to working out at a particular time and place, you'll have a greater chance of meeting your goals," Dr. Rippe says. Try taking an aerobics class during your lunch hour, for example, or enjoy a brisk walk after dinner.

Find an exercise partner. Work out with a friend who's at a similar fitness level, Dr. Snell suggests.

Vary your activities. Walk on Monday, cycle on Wednesday, play a round of golf on Sunday, and so forth. If you walk regularly, give yourself a change of scenery by varying your route, Dr. Rippe advises. Should you grow weary of your regular Tuesday-night step class, drop in on that Friday-night funk aerobics class that you've been meaning to try.

If you head outdoors, adapt to the weather. "In cold weather, dress in layers that you can remove as your body heats up," Dr. Rippe says. In warm weather, he says, wear loose clothing and drink lots of water before and during your workout. In stormy weather, try walking on an indoor track at the health club or at the mall.

Add more movement to your day. At work, you might forgo your midmorning coffee break and go on a short walk instead. Or resolve to take the stairs instead of the elevator at least once a day.

Reward yourself for meeting your exercise goals. Buy a new shade of lipstick or a new tie. Splurge on some new workout gear. "Even a hot bath can be a reward," Dr. Rippe says.

CHAPTER NINE

Shed Those Extra Pounds

If you're trying to scale down your cholesterol, chances are good that you're trying to scale down, period. "Being 20 to 30 percent over your ideal weight and having high cholesterol frequently go hand in hand," says John W. Zamarra, M.D., founding director of the cardiac rehabilitation program at Placentia-Linda Community Hospital in Brea, California.

What's more, carrying excess pounds tends to deflate the body's level of "good" HDL cholesterol, the stuff that helps whisk "bad" LDL cholesterol out of the body. "People who are overweight generally have low HDL cholesterol, often accompanied by elevated total and LDL cholesterol," Dr. Zamarra says.

But chin up: Dropping those extra pounds can help you take control of your cholesterol. Even shedding a few pounds—5 to 10 percent of your initial weight—can significantly improve cholesterol levels, according to one study.

LOVE HANDLES? CHECK YOUR CHOLESTEROL

Numerous studies have made a connection between body weight, elevated cholesterol levels, and risk of coronary heart disease.

Using data from the second National Health and Nutrition Examination Survey, researchers from the University of Texas Southwestern Medical Center at Dallas Southwestern Medical School and other institutions examined the relationship between excess body weight and high blood cholesterol levels. These researchers conducted two separate studies—one with men, the other with women. Both reached the same conclusion: Excess body weight is associated with higher levels of total and LDL cholesterol and lower levels of HDL cholesterol in White men and women, whatever their ages. Perimenopausal and menopausal women had lower HDL cholesterol and higher total and LDL cholesterol levels than premenopausal women, regardless of their weight.

What's more, researchers discovered a stronger connection between body weight and triglyceride levels than between body weight and cholesterol. High levels of triglycerides (another type of blood fat) are now established as an independent risk factor for coronary heart disease in men and women, says William P. Castelli, M.D., medical director of the Framingham Cardiovascular Institute, a wellness program at Metro West Medical Center in Massachusetts.

Losing weight is one thing; keeping it off is quite another. But it can be done. Refer to the previous two chapters to learn more about avoiding cholesterol-raising foods and getting enough exercise, and follow these tips to help shed pounds permanently.

Work that body. There's no way around it, experts say. "The only way to lose weight is to burn more calories than you consume—not just today or this week, but on a regular basis," says Leonard Doberne, M.D., an endocrinologist in Mount View, California.

More important, regular exercise can maintain or even raise HDL cholesterol. While cutting back on dietary fat and cholesterol can often lower total blood cholesterol levels about 15 percent, it also tends to reduce HDL cholesterol, notes Dr. Doberne. "So the ratio of total cholesterol to HDL cholesterol, which appears to be of primary importance, is not always much improved," he says. "Exercise is the best way we know to raise HDL. That's why a weight-loss program aimed at improving the cholesterol ratio should include exercise."

Avoid crash diets. They tend to slow the metabolism until the body kicks into survival mode and starts storing fat like crazy, says Peg Jordan, R.N., in her book *How the New Food Labels Can Save Your Life*. Worse, once you start eating normally again, your metabolism is still sluggish, so any pounds you may have lost quickly return.

Think twice about high-protein diets. Many people who once devoured pretzels and bagels—both laden with carbohydrates—have given them up in favor of high-protein foods like beef. These diets are all based on the incorrect notion that carbohydrates make you fat. When people lose weight on a high-protein diet, they think it's because they're eating fewer carbohydrates, but it's really because they're eating fewer calories.

That said, high-protein diets vary in their approaches.

Some, like the Atkins Induction diet, popularized in *Dr. Atkins' New Diet Revolution,* literally drip with artery-clogging saturated fat. And they lack the health-protective benefits of vegetables, fruits, and whole grains. That in turn can lead to a jump in your cholesterol—and not the good HDL either.

There are some moderate high-protein diets, however, that have you cut back on starchy carbohydrates and sweets, substituting meat and tons of vegetables in their place. For most of us, that means swapping nutrient-empty white flour and sugar for nutrient-full protein and produce. So if you're going to go high-protein, better bets are *Sugar Busters!* and Dr. Barry Sears's *The Zone,* which focus on heart-healthy lean meat, poultry, fish, and low-fat cheese, which are all low in saturated fat.

Cut the fat. Eating fatty foods such as processed lunchmeat, fried snacks, and butter is the fastest route to weight gain, says Dr. Zamarra. "Fat contains 9 calories per gram, more than twice as many as carbohydrates and protein, which have only 4. You don't have to eat a lot of fatty foods to consume lots of calories."

Eat more complex carbohydrates. Specifically, choose whole grains, legumes, vegetables, and fruits, recommends dietitian Deralee Scanlon, R.D., author of *Diets That Work.*

Why? Because the body expends more calories digesting and metabolizing complex carbohydrates. To transform 100 calories of carbohydrates into stored body fat, the body must use 23 calories. But the body uses only 3 calories to convert 100 calories of dietary fat into body fat.

Foods high in complex carbohydrates tend to be higher in fiber and lower in calories and fat. It's likely that these foods also are more filling and take longer to chew—two qualities that can help you reduce the amount you eat.

Slow down. It takes about 20 minutes for your brain to let your body know that you've eaten enough, Scanlon says. If you eat quickly, you're likely to eat more than you really need.

If you rush through your meals like the cartoon Road Runner, Dr. Zamarra suggests that you try eating in a calm, settled atmosphere. A noisy, frenzied environment tends to make you eat faster—and more. Also, before you pick up your fork, close your eyes and take a few deep breaths. "This can help you eat at a slower, more leisurely pace," he says.

CHAPTER TEN

Soothe Your Stress

The hassles and headaches of everyday life eventually catch up with all of us. But chronic stress can give you more than just an urge to escape to a quiet South Seas island.

Although "it's not nearly as important a factor as diet," stress does have an effect on cholesterol levels as well as other risk factors for heart disease, says Dean Ornish, M.D., president and director of the Preventive Medicine Research Institute in Sausalito, California, and author of *Dr. Dean Ornish's Program for Reversing Heart Disease.*

When you react to stress with a fight-or-flight response—the same alert system that helped our caveman ancestors outrun predators—your body releases stress hormones such as cortisol and adrenaline into your bloodstream. These hormones speed up your breathing, increase your heart rate, and accelerate the flow of blood to your arms and legs (the better to help you flee). But if your body triggers this inner alarm dozens of times a day, it can lay the foundation for heart disease.

"Stress seems to accelerate the depositing of plaque into the arteries independent of its effect on blood cholesterol," Dr. Ornish says. In other words, stress causes harm not only through its effect on cholesterol but also through its effect on the arteries themselves.

"Stress can make your arteries constrict, which can reduce bloodflow to the heart," Dr. Ornish says. "It can cause something called plaque hemorrhage, which is a rupture of the lining of the arteries that can lead to obstruction of the arteries. And stress can cause blood to clot faster, which can lead to a heart attack."

THE SCIENCE BEHIND STRESS

Several years ago, a well-known study demonstrated that accountants' blood cholesterol skyrocketed by as many as 100 points above their usual levels during tax season. Another study showed that students' blood cholesterol spiked during exams.

Researchers at the University of Pittsburgh had 44 healthy men and women either take a complicated computerized test to raise their stress levels or rest quietly for 20 minutes. Blood samples were drawn before and after the test and the rest period. Those who took the test showed significant increases in total and "bad" LDL cholesterol.

And in Israel, researchers studied 104 men between the ages of 24 and 68. These men didn't have cardiovascular disease, but they did have highly stressful jobs and were identified by the researchers as "burned out." (The study defined burnout as a mix of physical fatigue, mental exhaustion, and other symptoms.) After controlling for age, weight, and other factors, the researchers discovered that the total cholesterol of the most burned-out men was 14 percent higher than that of the most relaxed men. What's more, the most stressed-out men had significantly higher LDL cholesterol, the kind that wreaks the most cardiovascular damage.

LEARNING TO LET GO

The bad news: There's no way to avoid stress. The good news: You can cope with stress in a more heart-healthy manner, experts say. "The impact of emotional stress has little to do with what's actually causing the stress and everything to do with how well you tolerate it," says David Bresler, Ph.D., a stress and imagery specialist at the Los Angeles Healing Arts Center. "Some people experience minimal stress and fall apart, while others face serious stress and don't have a problem with it."

So if you're following a low-fat, low-cholesterol diet and making other lifestyle changes that lower your risk of heart disease, why not learn to outsmart stress, too?

Before you come apart at the seams the next time you're stuck in traffic . . . on your way to a wedding . . . perhaps *your* wedding, consider your cholesterol level and try these stress-busting tips.

- Breathe deeply. "Your breathing is a reflection of your mental state. It's a bridge between your mind and your body, and it can be used to change your frame of mind," Dr. Ornish says. "If you're feeling anxious, your breathing becomes more rapid and shallow. But consciously making yourself breathe more slowly and deeply can help calm you."

STRIKE A POSE . . . AND RELAX

More and more Americans are embracing yoga, a form of active meditation that originated in India 4,000 years ago, to banish back pain, relieve arthritis, and increase their strength and flexibility. Others are using it as a natural tranquilizer to help soothe emotional stress.

"Practicing yoga can help you enter what some people call an inner state, in which the mind becomes more tranquil," says Michael Lee, director of Phoenix Rising Yoga Therapy in Housatonic, Massachusetts. Westerners are most familiar with hatha yoga, which focuses on breathing and on assuming a series of poses, or *asanas*.

If you think you have to twist yourself into a pretzel to reap the physical and mental benefits of yoga, think again. "Yoga postures can be very uncomplicated," says Christine Kaur, a yoga instructor in Los Angeles who has taught the discipline for more than 20 years. "But even the simplest postures can produce tremendous health benefits."

Some studies have shown that stress-management techniques such as yoga can reduce cholesterol levels, according to Dean Ornish, M.D., president and director of the Preventive Medicine Research Institute in Sausalito, California. Dr. Ornish includes the practice of yoga techniques, including breathing, meditation, visualization, and progressive relaxation, in his program for people with heart disease.

How to Do It

Interested in exploring the benefits of yoga for yourself? Consider enrolling in a yoga class, suggests Lee. To find a class, check the yellow pages under "Yoga Instruction" or see if your local YM/YWCA offers classes. Before you sign up, though, make sure the instructor emphasizes yoga as a form of relaxation rather than as a form of spiritual enlightenment or rigorous exercise. Lee suggests sitting in on a class or two so that you can see the class—and the instructor—in action.

"Find an instructor you feel compatible with," Lee suggests. "Avoid instructors who believe that yoga has to 'hurt to work' or who are very results-oriented and believe that you have to reach a certain level of achievement." Choosing the right yoga class is like trying on clothing—you have to see what fits.

In the meantime, Lee suggests the following simple stress-relieving exercise.

1. While standing or sitting, place your arms behind your back and clasp your hands. If your hands don't meet comfortably, "cheat" by holding the ends of a towel.

2. Move your arms upward and outward. Feel the stretch across your chest (but don't go so far that it hurts).

3. Take a deep breath. As you exhale, continue to stretch, opening up your chest and keeping your hands clasped.

4. Continue to take full, deep breaths, drawing air down into your belly and letting it out again. After several minutes, take one more breath and slowly unclasp your hands.

• **Get some exercise.** According to experts, aerobic exercise, such as a brisk stroll, can help reduce the amount of stress-producing hormones barreling through your bloodstream. "Exercise is a great stress-reducing tool," says Peter O. Kwiterovich, Jr., M.D., professor of medicine and director of the Lipid Research and Atherosclerosis Unit at Johns Hopkins University School of Medicine in Baltimore and author of *The Johns Hopkins Complete Guide for Preventing and Reversing Heart Disease.* "I recommend regular aerobic exercise. Try to be active ½ hour a day, three or four times a week."

• **Don't spread yourself too thin**—it's a major cause of stress, says James W. Anderson, M.D., professor of medicine and clinical nutrition at the University of Kentucky College of Medicine in Lexington. "Schedule your time carefully and learn to say no when you need to."

• **Try turning a stressful situation into a challenge,** Dr. Bresler suggests. "If your boss demands a report in two hours, for example, you can think, 'This isn't fair' or 'I might get fired if I don't do a good job,' " he says. Thinking this way can trigger fear and anger as well as the physiological responses associated with those emotions.

But if you choose to think, "This is a real challenge! Let's see what I can accomplish in two hours," you can transform negative stress into the positive kind. "You can wrap the identical situation in a completely different package, which will influence how your body responds," he says.

CHAPTER ELEVEN

Master Your Vices

Our society gives us the OK to enjoy certain products that we know aren't necessarily healthy for us, particularly when we consume too much of them. We're not talking about steaks and fatty cheeses here—we covered those in earlier chapters.

No, now it's time to talk about those other little vices that bring so many people a moment of pleasure: the calming cigarette, the relaxing glass of wine, and the eye-opening cup of coffee. All of these can affect your heart or cholesterol health in varying degrees and are worthy of discussion.

The good news is that even if your cholesterol is high, you may still be able to enjoy two of these habits—alcohol and coffee—in moderation. If you smoke, though, it's time to make a concerted effort to stop.

SMOKING

These days, smoking takes real willpower. If you smoke, chances are you're getting tired of enduring disdainful looks from coworkers who see you standing outdoors on a cigarette break. Or you feel frustrated trying to find restaurants that still have smoking sections. But feeling like a social outcast can't begin to match the havoc that smoking can wreak on your cholesterol levels—and the health of your heart. If you need even more reasons to quit, consider these two facts.

• If you smoke, you're more than twice as likely as a nonsmoker to have a heart attack. That's because cigarette smoke oxidizes LDL cholesterol (the "bad" stuff), making it more likely to form artery-clogging plaque. Motivate yourself to banish the butts with the knowledge that within 2 years of quitting, your risk of heart attack drops to the level of someone who never smoked at all.
• Smokers tend to have less HDL cholesterol (the "good" kind) and higher total and LDL than nonsmokers.

Scientists still aren't sure exactly how and why smoking is responsible for elevated cholesterol. Researchers in Turkey, however, studied 58 men (27 who smoked and 31 who did not), measuring the activity of lecithin cholesterol acyltransferase (LCAT), a key factor in shepherding cholesterol to the liver for excretion from the body. The researchers found that smoking affected HDL cholesterol levels and that LCAT activity tended to be lower in smokers than in nonsmokers, suggesting a correlation between smoking and LCAT.

A similar study, conducted by investigators at the University of California, Berkeley, found that the effectiveness of LCAT is "dramatically inhibited" by cigarette smoke. "Cigarette smoke hits human plasma with a double whammy" and reduces both LCAT and HDL, says Mark R. McCall, Ph.D., one of the researchers.

Research has shown that smoking also accelerates hardening of the arteries (arteriosclerosis) and leaves fatty deposits on artery walls (atherosclerosis). Further, cigarette smoke increases the level of carbon monoxide in the blood. This poisonous chemical robs cells of oxygen, injuring the lining of the arteries, and allowing fatty material to pass from the bloodstream into the vessel walls.

It's Never Too Late to Quit

"If you smoke, quitting is almost certainly the best thing that you can do for your cardiovascular system and for your overall health and quality of life," says John W. Zamarra, M.D., founding director of the cardiac rehabilitation program at Placentia-Linda Community Hospital in Brea, California.

It *is* possible to quit, no matter how many times you've tried in the past. More than 3 million Americans quit smoking every year. Consider these suggestions and join their ranks.

• Keep a smoking journal for 2 weeks before you quit, suggest C. Richard Conti, M.D., and Diana Tonnessen in their book *Beating the Odds against Heart Disease and High Cholesterol.* Jot down the circumstances that most often prompt you to light up: during your coffee break, after dinner, while chatting on the phone, when you're feeling lonely or bored, and so forth.

• After a week, review your journal, pinpointing circumstances that prompt you to smoke. Then list alternatives to lighting up during those times. If your journal shows that you tend to smoke after meals, for example, brush your teeth or take a walk instead.

• Decide whether you want to quit smoking all at once— that is, "cold turkey"—or taper off. While you may decide to stop smoking gradually, there's evidence that most successful quitters go cold turkey.

• Get a buddy to help you make it through the quitting process. This person can be a nonsmoker, a former smoker, or a smoker who will quit with you. Call your buddy when the going gets rough.

• Pick a "quit day" and mark it on your calendar. Make it no later than 1 week away. Many experts suggest quitting on a weekend, when most people have better control of their time, surroundings, and circumstances.

• Tell your family, friends, and coworkers about your quit day. Letting people know about your decision to quit smoking will help hold you to your resolve.

• Call or write your local chapter of the American Heart Association, the American Cancer Society, or the American Lung Association, and ask for their free brochures and pamphlets on smoking cessation.

• Get some kind of exercise. "Women who work out are conscious of their health and tend not to smoke," says Myra Muramoto, M.D., assistant professor of family and community medicine and medical director of the Arizona Program for Nicotine and Tobacco Research at the University of Arizona in Tucson.

• Consider buproprion (Zyban), a prescription antidepressant approved as a smoking-cessation aid. In one study, researchers from the Arizona Program for Nicotine and Tobacco Research found that almost two times as many smokers who took Zyban were able to abstain from tobacco as those who used either nicotine patches or an inactive placebo.

• Throw away all of your cigarettes and matches. Soak the cigarettes in water so that you can't scrounge them out of the trash.

• Hide all the ashtrays. Better yet, get rid of them.

• Lay in a supply of healthy snacks such as celery, carrots, apples, sunflower seeds, and air-popped popcorn. They'll keep your mouth and fingers busy without wreaking havoc on your shape.

• Take a long walk or visit a nonsmoking environment such as a library, museum, or movie theater.

• Plan to have your teeth cleaned to get rid of tobacco stains. Resolve to keep them that way.

• Avoid stressful situations and smoking environments (bars, for example). Spend as much time as possible in places where smoking isn't permitted.

Staying Smoke-Free

What about withdrawal symptoms? About 80 percent of smokers experience symptoms when they quit, ranging from headaches and fatigue to nausea, diarrhea, and constipation. Some people also feel anxious, depressed, or irritable or have trouble sleeping. Withdrawal symptoms, however, tend to subside in 2 to 3 days, after the nicotine has left your body, and will be gone—or nearly so—within a couple of weeks.

Here are three ways to kick the habit for good.

• Be alert for "smoke signals." One study identified the four most likely relapse scenarios: during social drinking, after a meal, while feeling anxious at work, and while feeling depressed or anxious when at home alone.

• Learn a relaxation technique, such as deep breathing or guided imagery. If smoking helps you relax, "you're likely to feel more tense when you quit smoking unless you have other ways to manage stress that don't revolve around cigarettes," says Dean Ornish, M.D., president and director of the Preventive Medicine Research Institute in Sausalito, California, and author of *Dr. Dean Ornish's Program for Reversing Heart Disease.*

• On an index card, list two or three of your most important reasons for quitting smoking. Stash the card in your pocket or purse, or wherever you used to keep your cigarettes. Pull it out and go over the list often, particularly when you feel the urge to smoke.

ALCOHOL

Drinking protects your heart, right?

Not necessarily.

But that's the message some Americans came away with several years ago when a few studies indicated that moderate drinking is associated with reduced risk of coronary heart disease. The truth is, deciding whether to imbibe to protect your heart isn't as simple as deciding to eat less saturated fat and more soluble fiber.

On the one hand, there's evidence that moderate consumption of alcohol can help reduce the risk of coronary heart disease as well as help raise levels of "good" HDL cholesterol. On the other hand, many experts question the wisdom of encouraging people to drink for their health. In fact, some health professionals suggest that the decision to drink moderately for health purposes be made with the guidance of a physician.

Experts do agree on another point: If you don't drink, don't start.

The following facts can help you make an informed decision about the benefits—and risks—of moderate drinking to raise HDL and lower heart disease risk.

The Benefits of Limited Consumption

Moderate alcohol consumption seems to beneficially raise HDL cholesterol, but experts aren't sure why. "We don't entirely understand the effect of alcohol on HDL," says Peter O. Kwiterovich Jr., M.D., professor of medicine and director of the Lipid Research and Atherosclerosis Unit at Johns Hopkins University School of Medicine in Baltimore. "But it's pretty clear from epidemiological studies that people who drink moderately do better than people who don't drink at all."

"The data are clear that a drink or two a day lowers heart attack risk," agrees William P. Castelli, M.D., medical director of the Framingham Cardiovascular Institute, a wellness program at Metro West Medical Center in Massachusetts.

According to data from the second National Health and Nutrition Examination Survey, average levels of HDL cholesterol were higher among drinkers than among abstainers, no matter what their age, sex, or race.

And for 7 years, the Multiple Risk Factor Intervention Trial followed a subgroup consisting of 11,688 middle-aged men who were at high risk for heart disease. During that time, those who consumed about two drinks per day (with each drink equal to 4 ounces of wine, 12 ounces of beer, or 1 ½ ounces of 80-proof spirits) had higher HDL levels than nondrinkers. This alcohol intake seemed largely responsible for a 22 percent reduced chance of death from heart disease, researchers said.

In one of Dr. Kwiterovich's studies, he and his colleagues had 56 men with low levels of HDL either drink one beer a day or abstain from alcohol. After 2 months, there were no differences in HDL levels between the two groups. But the beer drinkers did experience a 10 percent increase in apolipoprotein A-1, the major protein component of HDL. This protein is believed to help extract cholesterol from the cells and move it to the liver for excretion.

Not a Magic Bullet

If you think that simply hoisting a beer stein or sipping your favorite Bordeaux will fix your cholesterol levels, think again. "Two glasses of wine a day will have a modest effect on your HDL, and even that modest effect is beneficial," Dr. Castelli says. "But if you're looking for a magic bullet, this isn't it."

Further, overimbibing to benefit your cholesterol can be risky, experts say. "Alcohol is like coffee—it has some theoretical benefits and some potential risks," says Neal Barnard, M.D., president of the Physicians Committee for Responsible Medicine in Washington, D.C.

Those risks include developing certain cancers and provoking cardiac arrhythmias and cirrhosis of the liver, says Dr. Castelli.

"It appears that women have an increased risk of breast cancer from increased alcohol consumption, even at the moderate levels recommended as potentially beneficial for heart disease," says Marla Mendelson, M.D., assistant professor of medicine at Northwestern University Medical School in Chicago. "So women who have other risk factors for breast cancer must think twice about drinking."

There are other issues to consider. "If you have high blood pressure, alcohol can raise it more," says Frederic J. Pashkow, M.D., a cardiologist at the Cleveland Clinic Foundation in Ohio and author of *50 Essential Things to Do When the Doctor Says It's Heart Disease.*

What's more, alcohol can actually raise triglycerides, another blood fat implicated in heart disease, by lowering the concentration of an enzyme used to break them down. "Even having a glass of wine with dinner every night can substantially raise triglycerides in people who are overweight or who have hereditary triglyceride problems," says Thomas Bersot, M.D., associate professor of medicine at the University of California, San Francisco.

The bottom line? If you choose to imbibe, do so in moderation—and if you don't drink, don't start, says Margo Denke, M.D., associate professor of medicine in the Center for Human Nutrition at the University of Texas Southwestern Medical Center at Dallas.

Dr. Barnard agrees. "I suggest that people follow a low-fat diet. I'm not sure that adding alcohol to that would be helpful."

COFFEE

Whether you linger over designer lattes at trendy coffee bars or savor fresh, strong joe from your trusty old percolator, one thing's for sure: When it comes to the relationship between coffee consumption and elevated blood cholesterol, there's controversy brewing.

Some studies suggest that coffee can raise cholesterol levels; others conclude just the opposite. Most of the studies conducted in the United States have found that people who don't drink coffee have higher rates of coronary heart disease than coffee drinkers. In fact, the prestigious Framingham Heart Study concluded that drinking up to five cups of coffee a day may actually have lowered the risk of coronary heart disease, Dr. Castelli says.

The good news is that consuming moderate amounts of coffee does not appear to raise the risk of heart disease. What's more, some experts say that a cup or two of coffee a day shouldn't significantly affect your cholesterol level. (No large studies have been conducted on the effect of other caffeinated foods or drinks—such as chocolate or cola—on blood cholesterol levels.)

But caffeine can affect the body in other ways. Consumed in large amounts, it can sap bone strength and accelerate heart rate. Further complicating the coffee/cholesterol issue is the role of nicotine. Some studies note that avid coffee drinkers tend to smoke more than people who drink coffee in moderate amounts, and smoking has definitely been implicated in the development of coronary heart disease.

Also, "caffeine tends to stimulate hunger in certain people," says Connie Diekman, R.D., a dietitian in St. Louis and a spokesperson for the American Dietetic Association. "Some people may respond by eating foods that increase their cholesterol levels. But it's difficult to isolate the effect of caffeine on cholesterol and to determine whether the increases in cholesterol are caused by caffeine or by something else."

The Caffeine/Cholesterol Connection

Investigators have conducted numerous studies on the relationship between coffee, elevated cholesterol, and heart disease. Results have been inconclusive, however. Some of these studies show that when it comes to coffee and cholesterol, much depends on how the coffee is prepared, according to Dr. Castelli. "Boiled coffee, like the kind drunk in Scandinavia and Turkey, tends to raise cholesterol and the risk of heart disease," Dr. Castelli says. Filtered coffee, however, doesn't increase the risk of heart disease.

Researchers at Johns Hopkins Medical Institutions in Baltimore had 100 healthy men drink varying amounts of filtered coffee each day: 24 ounces of regular coffee, 12 ounces of regular coffee, 24 ounces of decaffeinated coffee, or no coffee at all. After 8 weeks, the men who drank the 24 ounces of regular coffee a day experienced small increases in their total cholesterol, because of slight rises in their "bad" LDL and "good" HDL cholesterol. The researchers concluded that these small increases in LDL and HDL together "should not affect coronary heart disease risk." That's because small changes in HDL can protect against much larger changes in LDL, Dr. Castelli explains.

But some research does reinforce the need for moderation. Researchers at Boston University polled 858 women hospitalized with a first heart attack and an equal number of healthy women on their health habits, including coffee consumption. Researchers found that compared with non–coffee drinkers, women who said they drank five to six cups of coffee a day had a 40 percent greater risk of a heart attack; women who drank seven to nine cups, a 70 percent greater risk. But women who drank less than five cups of coffee a day had no higher risk than women who didn't drink coffee at all.

Enjoy Coffee—But Watch the Lattes

Most people don't have to be overly anxious about their caffeine intakes, says Robert J. Nicolosi, Ph.D., director of the Center for Cardiovascular Disease Control at the University of Lowell in Massachusetts. "In my view, avoiding caffeine is not one of the lifestyle interventions you need to be most concerned about."

Diekman concurs. "If you enjoy coffee in moderation and it's not affecting your body—such as accelerating your heart rate—continue to drink it," she says. "But keep in mind that coffee provides no nutritional value. So make sure it's not crowding nourishing beverages (such as juice or fat-free milk) out of your diet."

If, however, you are at high risk for heart attack, some experts would advise that you make sure you drink less than four cups a day. And while it's not certain whether caffeine can harm a developing fetus, mothers-to-be should avoid caffeine during their entire pregnancies, recommends Evelyn Tribole, R.D., a dietitian in Beverly Hills, California, and author of *Healthy Homestyle Cooking*.

And take care with flavored and specialty coffees, including those served at the local coffee bar, says Barbie Casselman, a nutrition consultant in Toronto. Some coffee beverages contain large amounts of high-fat milk and syrup, so you may be sipping more fat and calories than you realize.

"Most people think that a cappuccino is 6 ounces of coffee and 2 ounces of whipped milk," Casselman says. "But a regular-size cappuccino is actually 2 ounces of espresso plus a cup of milk; a large cappuccino has 12 ounces of milk. If it's whole milk, you might be consuming about 200 calories and 8 grams of fat in 12 ounces. You could eat a dessert for that!"

PART IV

The Outsmart Cholesterol Food Guide

CHAPTER TWELVE

The Outsmart Cholesterol
14-Day Menu Planner

Want to enjoy three meals plus snacks each day and still lower your cholesterol? Have we got a menu plan for you!

This nutritionist-approved plan, designed specifically to help lower cholesterol, features meals and snacks that provide a total of about 2,000 calories a day, with 55 percent of calories from complex carbohydrates (starches), 20 percent from fat, 15 percent from protein, and 10 percent from simple carbohydrates (sugars). Of the 20 percent of calories from fat, only about 5 percent comes from saturated fat. In comparison, the typical American diet gets 13 percent of calories from saturated fat.

As for cholesterol, this plan allows 150 milligrams a day, which is half of the American Heart Association's recommended limit of 300 milligrams a day for people without coronary heart disease. The plan also contains more fiber and less sodium than the typical American diet. All meals provide one serving.

You can follow the menu plan exactly as listed here, adapt it to include your own healthy favorites, or replace some of the meal ideas with the delicious recipes in chapter 13. Keep in mind, though, that if you veer from the foods offered in the plan, your nutritional intake for the day—including total calories, fat calories, and milligrams of cholesterol—will probably change.

Also remember that, in the long run, the key to sticking with an eating plan that cuts cholesterol is to keep your meals not just healthy but varied, delicious, and fun.

Day I
Breakfast
¾ cup grape juice
I cup oatmeal with ¼ cup raisins and ¼ cup fat-free milk
⅛ wedge cantaloupe

Lunch
I cup cooked pasta with ½ cup low-sodium marinara sauce
Tossed salad: I cup chopped romaine lettuce, ½ cup shredded carrots, and ½ cup shredded red cabbage, dressed with 2 teaspoons canola oil, 2 tablespoons vinegar, and a dash of sweet basil
Garlic bread: 2 slices toasted Italian bread, brushed with 2 teaspoons olive oil and rubbed with I clove fresh garlic

Dinner
Fresh vegetable platter: ¼ cup cauliflower, ¼ cup chopped mushrooms, and ¼ green pepper, sliced
Vegetable dip: ¼ cup fat-free yogurt, flavored with I scallion, chopped

3 ounces broiled haddock
¾ cup steamed rice
1 cup steamed broccoli with ¼ teaspoon fresh ginger or
a dash of ground ginger
½ cup cubed winter squash and ¼ cup crushed pineapple, sprinkled with nutmeg

Snacks
2 ounces fat-free unsalted pretzels
1 apple, sliced and topped with ½ cup low-fat vanilla yogurt, 2 teaspoons wheat germ, and 1 tablespoon slivered
almonds
Daily totals: 1,932 calories, 34 g total fat, 3.6 g saturated
fat, 65 mg cholesterol, 30 g dietary fiber, 1,457 mg sodium

Day 2
Breakfast
½ English muffin with 1 tablespoon strawberry spread
and 1 teaspoon heart-healthy margarine
½ cup low-fat vanilla yogurt with 2 tablespoons wheat
germ
1 orange

Lunch
1 cup grape juice
Turkey sandwich: 1 ounce white meat turkey on 2 slices
whole wheat bread with lettuce, tomato, and 1 teaspoon
mustard
Tossed salad: 3 cups chopped greens, ¼ cup chickpeas,
and 1 carrot, sliced, dressed with 2 teaspoons olive oil
and 2 tablespoons flavored vinegar
4 graham crackers

Dinner

1 cup low-sodium minestrone soup

3 ounces lean roast beef

1 baked potato, topped with butter-flavored sprinkles and a dash of garlic powder

½ cup steamed Brussels sprouts, topped with 1 tablespoon vinegar and a dash of mustard powder

2 slices Italian bread with 2 teaspoons heart-healthy margarine

1 cup canned peaches, in juice

Snacks

½ bagel with 1 tablespoon low-fat cream cheese

1 pear

Daily totals: 1,982 calories, 36 g total fat, 9 g saturated fat, 96 mg cholesterol, 38 g dietary fiber, 1,796 mg sodium

Day 3
Breakfast

¾ cup orange juice

1 cup ready-to-eat raisin bran cereal with ½ cup fat-free milk

2 dried figs

Lunch

Vegetable burger on whole wheat bun with lettuce, tomato, onion, and mustard

½ cup commercially prepared three-bean salad

1 carrot and 1 rib celery, cut into sticks

½ cup low-fat coffee-flavored yogurt

1 tangerine or other fresh fruit

Dinner

Tossed salad: 3 cups chopped romaine lettuce, 2 slices tomato, 2 radishes, 2 slices cucumber, and ½ carrot, sliced, dressed with 2 teaspoons olive oil and 2 tablespoons vinegar

3 ounces grilled or baked chicken breast, rubbed with fresh garlic and ½ teaspoon olive oil

1 cup steamed brown rice

Savory cabbage: ½ cup shredded cabbage and ¼ cup chopped onions, sautéed in 2 teaspoons olive oil, ½ teaspoon savory, and ½ teaspoon dill

1 baked apple with 2 tablespoons maple syrup

Snacks

3 fat-free devil's food cookies

2 cups air-popped popcorn with ½ teaspoon butter-flavored sprinkles

Daily totals: 1,969 calories, 38 g total fat, 8.6 g saturated fat, 95 mg cholesterol, 39 g dietary fiber, 1,909 mg sodium

Day 4

Breakfast

1½ cups ready-to-eat multigrain cereal with ½ cup fat-free milk, sprinkled with 5 almonds, chopped

½ red grapefruit

Lunch

1 cup low-sodium split pea soup

1 toasted English muffin with 2 teaspoons heart-healthy margarine

¾ cup low-fat or fat-free strawberry yogurt with 1 teaspoon rice bran or wheat germ

Dinner

Pork stir-fry: 1 ounce lean pork loin, 1 cup sliced bok choy, ½ cup snow peas, ¼ cup diced red peppers, and ¼ cup diced celery, stir-fried in 1 teaspoon minced fresh garlic, 2 teaspoons canola oil, and a dash of sesame oil

1½ cups steamed brown rice with a dash of poultry seasoning or sage

Tossed salad: 1 cup shredded romaine lettuce, ¼ cup chopped red onions, and 2 radishes, dressed with 1 tablespoon lemon juice and 2 teaspoons olive oil

1 banana or other fresh fruit

Snacks

1 cup grapes

1 bake-and-eat soft pretzel (2½ ounces, baked without salt)

Daily totals: 1,941 calories, 40 g total fat, 6.8 g saturated fat, 33 mg cholesterol, 25 g dietary fiber, 1,465 mg sodium

Day 5

Breakfast

1 English muffin with 2 teaspoons heart-healthy margarine

Breakfast blender drink: 1 cup fat-free milk and ½ cup fresh or unsweetened frozen strawberries, blended until frothy

Lunch

Pita sandwich: 1 ounce cubed low-fat Cheddar cheese and ½ cup each chopped spinach, tomato, and onion, stuffed in a pita and dressed with 2 tablespoons fat-free dressing (your choice)

1 carrot and 1 rib celery, cut into sticks
1 cup low-fat yogurt (your choice)

Dinner

2 slices pizza (ask for only half the cheese)
Tossed salad: 3 cups chopped greens, ¼ cup broccoli, ¼ cup chickpeas, 1 tablespoon chopped onions, and ¼ tomato, sliced, dressed with 2 tablespoons fat-free dressing (your choice)
1 cup grapes

Snacks

2 cups cooked pasta with ½ cup low-sodium marinara sauce
2 unsalted pretzels (2 ounces)
1 banana
Daily totals: 1,899 calories, 28 g total fat, 7 g saturated fat, 50 mg cholesterol, 26 g dietary fiber, 2,473 mg sodium

Day 6
Breakfast

¾ cup orange juice
Egg substitute, scrambled with 1 tablespoon fat-free milk in a nonstick pan
1 potato, sliced and sautéed with 1 tablespoon heart-healthy margarine, 2 tablespoons chopped onions, and ½ clove fresh garlic, minced, in a nonstick pan
2 slices toasted whole wheat bread with 2 teaspoons fruit spread

Lunch

1 cup low-sodium lentil soup
Tossed salad: 3 cups chopped greens, ½ cup sliced car-

rots, and ¼ cup sliced onions, dressed with 2 teaspoons olive oil and 1 tablespoon vinegar
1 toasted English muffin

Dinner
Chicken fajita: 3 ounces chicken strips (prepared in a low-fat manner), ¼ cup mashed avocado, ¼ cup salsa, ¼ cup fat-free plain yogurt, 1½ teaspoons olive oil, 1 teaspoon lime juice, and 1 teaspoon fresh cilantro in 1 flour tortilla
1½ cups steamed brown rice, flavored with 2 table-spoons salsa and ⅛ teaspoon chopped jalapeño peppers
10 low-fat tortilla chips (1 ounce)

Snacks
1 cup fresh or canned chunked pineapple, in juice
1 carrot, cut into sticks, with ¼ cup commercially pre-pared fat-free herbed yogurt cheese
Daily totals: 1,902 calories, 45 g total fat, 7.3 g saturated fat, 77 mg cholesterol, 29 g dietary fiber, 1,717 mg sodium

Day 7
Breakfast
½ bagel with 1 tablespoon light cream cheese
1 cup low-fat vanilla yogurt with 2 teaspoons wheat germ
½ mango, cubed

Lunch
2 ounces scallops, ½ cup chopped mushrooms, ¼ cup sliced onions, ¼ cup chopped celery, and ¼ cup chopped green peppers, sautéed in 1 teaspoon sesame oil, 1 ta-blespoon low-sodium soy sauce, 1 teaspoon grated fresh ginger, and 1 clove fresh garlic, minced

2 cups steamed rice
1 fortune cookie

Dinner
2 cups low-sodium vegetable soup
Tossed salad: 1 ounce flaked water-packed tuna, 4 cups chopped romaine lettuce, 1/4 cup shredded carrots, and 1 radish, dressed with 1 teaspoon olive oil and 1 tablespoon vinegar
Baked pita crisps: 1 pita, brushed with 2 teaspoons olive oil and assorted herbs and spices then broiled and broken into pieces
1 cup fresh fruit (grapes, apples, and oranges)

Snacks
2 graham crackers with 1 tablespoon peanut butter and 1 cup fat-free milk
1 banana
Daily totals: 2,030 calories, 40 g total fat, 10 g saturated fat, 61 mg cholesterol, 25 g dietary fiber, 1,761 mg sodium

Day 8
Breakfast
3/4 cup orange juice
1 cup oatmeal with 1/4 cup raisins and 1/2 cup fat-free milk
1 slice toasted whole wheat bread with 1 teaspoon heart-healthy margarine and 1 tablespoon apple butter

Lunch
1 cup low-sodium tomato soup
1/4 to 1/2 cup commercially prepared three-bean salad (add 1/4 cup chopped red onions, basil, and 2 tablespoons red wine vinegar)

2 slices rye bread with 2 teaspoons heart-healthy margarine

1 peach, nectarine, or other fresh fruit

Dinner

Bulgur salad: 1 cup cooked bulgur; 2 tablespoons parsley; ½ tomato, chopped; and 1 teaspoon lemon juice

Broiled skinless chicken breast

1 potato, baked, with 2 tablespoons fat-free sour cream and 2 teaspoons heart-healthy margarine

1 cup chopped spinach, sautéed in 1 teaspoon olive oil, ¼ cup chopped onions, and 1 clove fresh garlic, minced

1 hard roll (2 ounces) with 1 tablespoon heart-healthy margarine

2 cups cubed watermelon or other fruit

Snacks

2 cups air-popped popcorn with butter-flavored sprinkles and 1 teaspoon Parmesan cheese

1 fresh fig

Daily totals: 1,968 calories, 41 g total fat, 7 g saturated fat, 84 mg cholesterol, 41 g dietary fiber, 1,850 mg sodium

Day 9
Breakfast

¾ cup ready-to-eat fortified oat cereal with ½ cup fat-free milk

1 sliced banana

Lunch

1 oat bran and raisin muffin (2 ounces)

1 cup low-fat yogurt (your choice)

1 orange, sliced

Dinner

1 cup low-sodium vegetable soup (add ¼ cup white beans and 1 clove fresh garlic, minced, if desired)

3 ounces baked flounder

¼ cup chopped cabbage, sautéed in 2 teaspoons canola oil and ground red pepper (to taste) and served over 1 cup steamed rice

1 slice cornbread with 2 teaspoons heart-healthy margarine

1 baked apple with ½ teaspoon cinnamon and 2 teaspoons brown sugar

Snacks

6 graham crackers with 1 tablespoon almond butter or peanut butter

½ cup fat-free milk

Daily totals: 1,748 calories, 33 g total fat, 4 g saturated fat, 68 mg cholesterol, 31 g dietary fiber, 1,273 mg sodium

Day 10

Breakfast

1 cup cooked oat bran cereal with 1 tablespoon rice bran or wheat germ

2 cups cubed honeydew, casaba, or other melon

Lunch

1 applesauce muffin (1 ounce) with 2 teaspoons heart-healthy margarine

½ cup 2% cottage cheese with 2 cups fresh fruit (your choice)

Dinner

1 cup low-sodium vegetable juice

1 cup low-sodium green pea soup

Spinach salad: 2 cups spinach, ¼ cup sliced mushrooms, ¼ cup chopped red onions, and 1 clove fresh garlic, minced, dressed with 2 teaspoons olive oil and 2 tablespoons vinegar
4 garlic breadsticks (4 ounces)

Snacks
2 fig bars
1 orange
Fresh vegetable plate: 1 cup carrot sticks and ½ cup broccoli florets
Vegetable dip: 2 tablespoons commercially prepared fat-free herbed yogurt cheese
Daily totals: 1,796 calories, 41 g total fat, 11 g saturated fat, 10 mg cholesterol, 44 g dietary fiber, 1,985 mg sodium

Day 11
Breakfast
1 cup hot cereal with 1 tablespoon wheat germ and 2 tablespoons maple syrup
Fruit compote: 2 tablespoons prunes, 2 tablespoons figs, and 2 tablespoons raisins, cooked in 2 tablespoons orange juice and 2 tablespoons water

Lunch
1 cup low-sodium turkey vegetable soup
Tossed salad: 4 cups chopped romaine lettuce, dressed with 2 teaspoons olive oil and 2 tablespoons vinegar
2 slices toasted whole wheat bread
1 cup low-fat yogurt (your choice)

Dinner
3 ounces pork medallions in tomato sauce, served over 1 cup egg noodles

1 ½ cups steamed green beans and chopped carrots
2 slices rye bread with 2 teaspoons heart-healthy margarine
Streusel apple: 1 apple, baked with 1 tablespoon low-fat flavored yogurt, ½ tablespoon oats, and 1 teaspoon brown sugar

Snack
2 ounces low-sodium pretzel chips with mustard
Daily totals: 1,996 calories, 41 g total fat, 7.2 g saturated fat, 122 mg cholesterol, 32 g dietary fiber, 1,721 mg sodium

Day 12
Breakfast
1 cup ready-to-eat bran cereal with ½ cup fat-free milk
2 slices toasted whole wheat bread with 2 teaspoons heart-healthy margarine
1 banana

Lunch
½ grapefruit
Pasta salad: 1 cup cooked pasta, 1 ounce water-packed tuna, ½ cup snow peas, ½ cup frozen or canned plain artichoke hearts, and 2 scallions, chopped, dressed with 1 tablespoon low-fat mayonnaise, 1 tablespoon vinegar, and fresh basil and parsley
1 slice pumpernickel bread with 2 teaspoons heart-healthy margarine

Dinner
Chicken kebabs: 2 ounces cooked, cubed chicken breast with ¼ pepper, ½ tomato, 5 mushrooms, and ⅓ onion,

all cut into chunks; marinated in 2 teaspoons olive oil, 2 teaspoons lemon juice, 2 teaspoons low-sodium soy sauce, 1 tablespoon chopped parsley, ¼ teaspoon red-pepper flakes, 1 clove fresh garlic, minced, and ¼ chile pepper, minced

1½ cups steamed brown and wild rice, tossed with thyme or parsley

1 frozen fruit bar

Snacks
1 cup grapes

1 oat bran and raisin muffin (2 ounces)

Daily totals: 1,895 calories, 33 g total fat, 5 g saturated fat, 65 mg cholesterol, 38 g dietary fiber, 2,065 mg sodium

Day 13
Breakfast
Four 4-inch buckwheat pancakes with 4 tablespoons maple syrup

Citrus salad: ¼ cup grapefruit sections and ½ cup orange sections

Lunch
Egg drop soup: 1 cup hot low-fat chicken stock with 2 tablespoons egg substitute

Chicken teriyaki with vegetables (low-fat, low-calorie frozen entrée)

1½ cups steamed brown rice with chives

Wonton chips: 3 wonton wrappers, misted with nonstick cooking spray and baked

3 kumquats or ½ cup fresh or canned chunked pineapple, in juice

Dinner

Omelette: ⅓ cup chopped mushrooms and ⅓ cup chopped onions, sautéed in 2 teaspoons olive oil and folded into ½ cup beaten egg substitute
2 slices toasted whole wheat bread with 2 teaspoons heart-healthy margarine and 1 tablespoon strawberry spread
1 apple, sliced, with 1 tablespoon natural peanut butter

Snacks

1 carrot, cut into sticks
2 slices melba toast with 1 ounce low-fat Swiss cheese
Daily totals: 1,805 calories, 42 g total fat, 11.4 g saturated fat, 123 mg cholesterol, 32 g dietary fiber, 1,978 mg sodium

Day 14

Breakfast
¾ cup tropical fruit juice
2 whole grain waffles, topped with ½ cup low-fat yogurt (your choice) and ½ cup blueberries

Lunch
Turkey sandwich: 1 ounce low-fat turkey breast lunchmeat and 1 ounce low-fat Swiss cheese on 2 slices rye bread with lettuce, tomato, and 2 teaspoons mustard
1 carrot, cut into sticks
Curry dip: ¼ cup fat-free plain yogurt and ¼ cup fat-free mayonnaise, blended with ½ teaspoon curry and 1 clove fresh garlic, minced

Dinner
3 ounces boneless, skinless chicken breast, poached with ¼ cup chopped onions, ¼ cup chopped carrots, and 1

tablespoon parsley and served over 1 cup steamed chopped spinach

Hawaiian rice: 1 cup cooked brown rice with ½ cup snow peas, 4 pieces baby corn, and ¼ cup water chestnuts; sautéed in 1 teaspoon peanut oil and ¼ teaspoon ground red pepper; and tossed with ¼ cup drained chunked pineapple

1 sweet potato, baked or steamed (top with cinnamon, if desired)

½ mango, sprinkled with ¼ cup macadamia nuts

Snack

1 slice cocoa angel food cake ($\frac{1}{12}$ cake) with ½ cup fresh raspberries

Daily totals: 2,108 calories, 53 g total fat, 11 g saturated fat, 101 mg cholesterol, 37 g dietary fiber, 2,228 mg sodium

CHAPTER THIRTEEN

Delicious Recipes That Outsmart Cholesterol

Who says you have to deprive yourself to control your cholesterol? The following recipes may look—and even better, taste—downright decadent, but they are actually good for you! We've removed cholesterol-boosting fat and added heart-healthy ingredients such as nuts, fruits, and vegetables for every meal of the day.

BREAKFASTS

Florentine Omelette
Hearty seasonings and a delicious medley of vegetables flavor this breakfast favorite.
2 eggs
2 egg whites
3 tablespoons water
1 teaspoon dried Italian seasoning, crushed
1/4 teaspoon salt
8 ounces mushrooms, sliced
1 onion, chopped

1 red bell pepper, chopped
1 clove garlic, minced
4 ounces (2 packed cups) spinach leaves, chopped
¾ cup (3 ounces) shredded low-fat mozzarella cheese

Preheat the oven to 200°F. Coat a baking sheet with cooking spray.

In a medium bowl, whisk together the eggs, egg whites, water, Italian seasoning, and salt.

Coat a large nonstick skillet with cooking spray and place over medium-high heat. Add the mushrooms, onion, pepper, and garlic and cook, stirring often, for 4 minutes, or until the pepper starts to soften. Add the spinach and cook for 1 minute, or until the spinach is wilted. Place in a small bowl and cover.

Wipe the skillet with a paper towel. Coat with cooking spray and place over medium heat. Pour in half of the egg mixture. Cook for 2 minutes, or until the bottom begins to set. Using a spatula, lift the edges to allow the uncooked mixture to flow to the bottom of the pan. Cook for 2 minutes longer, or until set. Sprinkle with half of the reserved vegetable mixture and half of the cheese. Cover and cook for 2 minutes, or until the cheese melts. Using a spatula, fold the egg mixture in half. Place on the prepared baking sheet and place in the oven to keep warm.

Coat the skillet with cooking spray. Repeat with the remaining egg mixture, vegetable mixture, and cheese to cook another omelette. To serve, cut each omelette in half.

Makes 4 servings

Per serving: 128 calories, 13 g protein, 7 g carbohydrates, 7 g total fat, 3 g saturated fat, 115 mg cholesterol, 3 g dietary fiber, 346 mg sodium

South-of-the-Border Frittata

Put eggs back on your menu with this Southwestern-inspired dish.

1 egg
5 egg whites
1 can (15 ounces) black beans, rinsed and drained
1 cup corn kernels
2/3 cup (2 1/2 ounces) shredded low-fat Monterey Jack cheese
3/4 teaspoon chili powder
1 bunch scallions, sliced
1/4 cup (2 ounces) fat-free sour cream
1/4 cup salsa

In a medium bowl, whisk together the egg, egg whites, beans, corn, cheese, and chili powder.

Coat a large nonstick skillet with cooking spray. Add the scallions. Coat lightly with cooking spray. Cook, stirring, over medium heat for 1 to 2 minutes, or until wilted.

Add the egg mixture to the skillet. Cook, stirring occasionally, for 7 to 8 minutes, or until the eggs are set on the bottom. Reduce the heat to low. Cover and cook for 4 to 5 minutes, or until the eggs are set on the top.

To serve, cut into wedges and top with the sour cream and salsa.

Makes 4 servings

Per serving: 229 calories, 20 g protein, 27 g carbohydrates, 6 g total fat, 3 g saturated fat, 67 mg cholesterol, 7 g dietary fiber, 751 mg sodium

Toasted Oat Muesli

Crunchy nuts and chewy dried fruit make this a filling start to any day.

6 cups old-fashioned oats, preferably thick-cut
1 1/4 cups sliced natural almonds

1 package (7 ounces) dried fruit bits
1 cup toasted wheat germ
½ cup unsalted raw pumpkin seeds
½ cup unsalted raw sunflower seeds

Preheat the oven to 325°F.

Spread the oats out on a jelly-roll pan. Spread the almonds in a small baking pan. Place the oats and almonds in the oven and bake, stirring often, until the oats are lightly browned and the almonds are toasted. The oats will take 30 to 35 minutes; the almonds will toast in 20 to 25 minutes.

Place the oats and almonds in a large bowl and cool completely.

Add the fruit bits, wheat germ, pumpkin seeds, and sunflower seeds. Toss to combine. Store in an airtight container.

To serve, place ½ cup of the cereal mixture in a bowl. Top with soy milk, fat-free milk, or yogurt.

Makes twenty-two ½-cup servings
Per serving: 300 calories, 12 g protein, 40 g carbohydrates, 11 g total fat, 1 g saturated fat, 0 mg cholesterol, 7 g dietary fiber, 2 mg sodium

Fruit and Nut Cereal

This fruit-sweetened cereal is rich in heart-healthy omega-3 fatty acids and disease-fighting fiber.

2 cups rolled oats
1 cup wheat flakes
2 tablespoons sunflower seeds
1½ tablespoons sesame seeds
¼ cup frozen apple juice concentrate, thawed
¼ cup packed brown sugar
2 tablespoons canola oil
½ teaspoon ground cinnamon

¼ cup chopped dried figs
¼ cup chopped dried apple rings
¼ cup chopped dried apricots
¼ cup slivered toasted almonds

Preheat the oven to 250°F. Coat a jelly-roll pan with cooking spray.

In a medium bowl, combine the oats, wheat flakes, sunflower seeds, sesame seeds, apple juice concentrate, brown sugar, oil, and cinnamon.

Spread the oat mixture in the prepared pan. Bake, stirring occasionally, for 45 to 60 minutes, or until golden brown. Cool completely.

Place the oat mixture, figs, apples, apricots, and almonds in an airtight container.

To serve, place ⅔ cup of the cereal mixture in a bowl. Top with soy milk, fat-free milk, or yogurt.

Makes about nine ⅔-cup servings
Per serving: 241 calories, 5 g protein, 40 g carbohydrates, 8 g total fat, 1 g saturated fat, 0 mg cholesterol, 4 g dietary fiber, 8 mg sodium

Multigrain Berry Waffles
The whole grain richness and sweet berries in these waffles turn a decadent treat into healthy eating.
1½ cups whole grain pastry flour
½ cup rolled oats
½ teaspoon baking powder
½ teaspoon baking soda
½ teaspoon salt
1⅔ cups fat-free milk
2 egg whites
3 tablespoons packed brown sugar
1 tablespoon vegetable oil

2 cups blueberries
1 ½ cups sliced strawberries
½ cup maple syrup

Preheat the oven to 200°F. Coat a baking sheet with cooking spray.

In a large bowl, combine the flour, oats, baking powder, baking soda, and salt.

In a medium bowl, combine the milk, egg whites, brown sugar, and oil. Add to the flour mixture and stir just until blended. Fold in 1 cup of the blueberries.

Coat a nonstick waffle iron with cooking spray. Preheat the iron.

Pour ½ cup of the batter onto the center of the iron. Cook for 5 minutes, or until steam no longer escapes from under the waffle-iron lid and the waffle is golden. Place the waffles on the prepared baking sheet and place in the oven to keep warm. Repeat with the remaining batter to make a total of 8 waffles.

Meanwhile, in a small saucepan over medium heat, combine the remaining 1 cup blueberries, the strawberries, and maple syrup. Cook for 5 minutes, or until the berries are softened and the mixture is hot. Serve with the waffles.

Makes 8 waffles
Per waffle: 239 calories, 7 g protein, 49 g carbohydrates, 3 g total fat, 0 g saturated fat, 1 mg cholesterol, 4 g dietary fiber, 217 mg sodium

Berry Berry Smoothie
Try this filling drink for a creamy fruit-flavored treat that's high in both vitamin C and fiber.
½ cup frozen unsweetened raspberries
½ cup frozen unsweetened strawberries
¾ cup unsweetened pineapple juice
1 cup soy milk or 1% milk

In a blender, combine the raspberries, strawberries, and pineapple juice. Add the milk and blend until smooth.

Makes 2 servings

Per serving: 102 calories, 4 g protein, 19 g carbohydrates, 3 g total fat, 0 g saturated fat, 0 mg cholesterol, 3 g dietary fiber. 16 mg sodium

SANDWICHES, SOUPS, AND SALADS

Grilled Vegetable Melts

These satisfying sandwiches are packed with healthy nutrients like calcium, folate, phosphorus, and vitamin A.

Basil Spread

1 cup packed fresh basil leaves
2 tablespoons grated Parmesan cheese
1 tablespoon toasted walnuts
1 clove garlic
¼ cup (2 ounces) fat-free cream cheese or sour cream

Sandwiches

2 zucchini, cut lengthwise into ¼"-thick slices
2 yellow and/or red bell peppers, quartered
1 red onion, cut crosswise into ¼"-thick slices
¼ teaspoon salt
1½ tablespoons balsamic vinegar
8 slices Italian bread, lightly toasted
4 slices low-fat Jarlsberg cheese

To make the basil spread: In a food processor, combine the basil, Parmesan, walnuts, and garlic. Process to puree. Add the cream cheese or sour cream. Process to mix. Set aside.

To make the sandwiches: Preheat the grill or broiler. Coat a grill rack or broiler-pan rack with cooking spray. Arrange the zucchini, peppers, and onion in a single layer on the prepared rack. Coat lightly with cooking spray. Sprinkle with the salt. Grill or broil for 10 minutes, turning once, or until lightly browned. Place on a plate and drizzle with the vinegar.

Arrange 4 of the bread slices on the rack. Spread with the basil mixture. Top with layers of zucchini, bell pepper, onion, and cheese. Grill or broil for 1 minute, or until the cheese melts. Top with the remaining bread slices.

Makes 4 servings

Per serving: 311 calories, 20 g protein, 46 g carbohydrates, 6 g total fat, 2 g saturated fat, 13 mg cholesterol, 5 g dietary fiber, 705 mg sodium

Niçoise Salad Pockets

This recipe is a great way to ease healthy flaxseed oil into your cholesterol-friendly diet.

Dressing

½ cup balsamic or cider vinegar
1 tablespoon extra-virgin olive oil
1 tablespoon flaxseed oil
1 teaspoon Dijon mustard
1 teaspoon dried Italian seasoning, crushed
1 clove garlic, minced

Sandwiches

¾ pound red potatoes, cut into ¼-thick slices
¼ pound small green beans
1 can (6 ounces) water-packed white tuna, drained and flaked
¼ red onion, thinly sliced
2 hard-cooked egg whites, coarsely chopped

¼ cup coarsely chopped niçoise olives
2 cups baby spinach leaves
4 whole wheat pitas, halved crosswise

To make the dressing: In a large bowl, combine the vinegar, olive oil, flaxseed oil, mustard, Italian seasoning, and garlic.

To make the sandwiches: Place a steamer basket in a saucepan with ½" of water. Place the potatoes and beans in the steamer. Bring to a boil over high heat. Reduce the heat to medium, cover, and cook for 7 minutes, or until crisp-tender. Rinse briefly under cold running water and drain.

To the bowl with the dressing, add the potatoes, beans, tuna, onion, egg whites, olives, and spinach. Toss to coat well.

Spoon the tuna mixture into each pita pocket. Drizzle lightly with any dressing left in the bowl.

Makes 4 servings
Per serving: 406 calories, 21 g protein, 56 g carbohydrates, 12 g total fat, 1 g saturated fat, 18 mg cholesterol, 9 g dietary fiber, 633 mg sodium

Minestrone Verde
This one-bowl meal is brimming with beans, pasta, and tender vegetables.
2 teaspoons extra-virgin olive oil
2 small leeks, white and green parts, halved lengthwise, rinsed, and thinly sliced
2 large ribs celery with leaves, thinly sliced
2 cloves garlic, minced + 1 whole clove garlic, peeled
¼ teaspoon dried oregano, crushed
¼ teaspoon freshly ground black pepper
⅛ teaspoon salt
2 cups water
1 cup chicken broth

　　4 cups chopped Swiss chard
　　⅔ cup frozen baby lima beans
　　¼ cup ditalini or other small pasta
　　¼ cup chopped Italian parsley
　　½ cup frozen green peas
　　4 teaspoons shredded Parmesan cheese

Heat the oil in a large saucepan over medium heat. Add the leeks, celery, minced garlic, oregano, pepper, and salt. Cook, stirring frequently, for 4 minutes, or until the vegetables begin to soften.

Add the water, broth, Swiss chard, lima beans, and pasta. Bring to a boil over high heat. Reduce the heat to medium-low, cover, and simmer for 8 minutes, or until the vegetables are tender and the pasta is al dente.

Meanwhile, coarsely chop the remaining garlic clove, then mince it together with the parsley. Stir the garlic-parsley mixture and the peas into the soup. Cover and cook for 5 minutes, or until the peas are heated through.

Ladle the soup into 4 bowls and top each with 1 teaspoon of the cheese.

Makes 4 servings

Per serving: 145 calories, 6 g protein, 24 g carbohydrates, 3 g total fat, 1 g saturated fat, 1 mg cholesterol, 5 g dietary fiber, 413 mg sodium

Gingery Vegetable Broth with Tofu and Noodles

Smoked tofu is available at many health food stores and keeps well.

　　1 tablespoon canola oil
　　8 ounces cremini mushrooms, finely chopped
　　2 large carrots, finely chopped
　　2 ribs celery, finely chopped

1 medium onion, finely chopped
6 large cloves garlic, minced
2 tablespoons finely chopped fresh ginger
3 tablespoons dry sherry
4 cups low-sodium vegetable broth
1/4 teaspoon salt
1 cup snow peas, cut into julienne strips
4 ounces thin soba noodles, broken in half
8 ounces baked smoked tofu, cut into 1/4 cubes
4 scallions, thinly sliced on the diagonal

Heat the oil in a large saucepan or Dutch oven over medium-high heat. Add the mushrooms, carrots, celery, onion, garlic, and ginger and cook, stirring often, for 10 minutes, or until the vegetables are lightly browned.

Add the sherry and cook for 1 minute, stirring to loosen browned bits from the pan. Add the broth and salt and bring to a boil over high heat. Reduce the heat to low, cover, and simmer for 45 minutes, adding the snow peas during the last 3 minutes.

Meanwhile, prepare the soba noodles according to package directions. Drain and set aside.

Stir the tofu, soba noodles, and scallions into the broth and simmer for 3 minutes, or until heated through.

Makes 4 servings
Per serving: 297 calories, 17 g protein, 40 g carbohydrates, 8 g total fat, 2 g saturated fat, 5 mg cholesterol, 6 g dietary fiber, 575 mg sodium

Mushroom-Barley Soup
Dried mushrooms help add a rich, meaty taste to the chicken broth of this soup. If you want to reduce fat even further, use one of the fat-free or reduced-fat broths available in stores.

1 ounce dried mushrooms
3 cups boiling water
4 carrots, chopped
2 large onions, chopped
2 ribs celery, chopped
12 ounces cremini or button mushrooms, stems removed,
sliced
1½ teaspoons dried oregano, crushed
5 cups chicken broth
1 cup barley
¼ teaspoon salt

Place the dried mushrooms in a small bowl and cover with the water. Let stand for 15 minutes.

Meanwhile, coat a large saucepan or Dutch oven with cooking spray. Add the carrots, onions, and celery. Coat lightly with cooking spray and set over medium heat. Cook, stirring occasionally, for 3 minutes. Add the sliced mushrooms and oregano. Cook, stirring occasionally, for 6 minutes, or until the vegetables are soft. Add the broth, barley, and salt. Cook for 10 minutes.

Line a sieve with a coffee filter or paper towel. Strain the dried mushroom water into the pot. Remove and discard the filter or paper towel. Rinse the dried mushrooms under running water to remove any grit. Chop and add to the pot.

Cook for 20 minutes, or until the barley is tender.

Makes 6 servings
Per serving: 185 calories, 8 g protein, 39 g carbohydrates, 1 g total fat, 0 g saturated fat, 0 mg cholesterol, 9 g dietary fiber, 628 mg sodium

Roasted Beet Salad
Oven roasting is a wonderful way to bring out the natural sweetness in beets.
4 medium beets (about 1 pound), stems trimmed to 1"

2 tablespoons apricot all-fruit spread
1 tablespoon white balsamic vinegar
1½ teaspoons olive oil
1½ teaspoons flaxseed oil
2 tablespoons snipped fresh chives or thinly sliced scallion
greens
½ teaspoon salt
¼ teaspoon freshly ground black pepper
2 medium navel oranges
4 cups mixed bitter salad greens, such as arugula, water-
cress, endive, and escarole

Preheat the oven to 400°F. Coat a 9" baking pan with cooking
spray.

Place the beets in the prepared baking pan and cover tightly
with foil. Roast for 1 hour, or until very tender. Uncover and
let the beets stand until cool enough to handle.

Meanwhile, in a large bowl, whisk the all-fruit spread, vinegar, olive oil, flaxseed oil, chives or scallions, salt, and pepper.

Slip the skins off the beets and discard the skins. Chop the
beets. Cut off the peel and white pith from the oranges. Section
the oranges into the bowl with the dressing. Add the beets and
toss to coat well. Let stand for at least 15 minutes to allow the
flavors to blend.

Just before serving, arrange the greens on a serving plate.
Top with the beet mixture.

Makes 4 servings

Per serving: 144 calories, 3 g protein, 27 g carbohydrates, 4 g
total fat, 0 g saturated fat, 0 mg cholesterol, 5 g dietary fiber,
390 mg sodium

Spinach Salad with Orange-Ginger Dressing
Prepare and refrigerate this dressing up to 3 days ahead,
if you like, so the final assembly becomes even easier.

2 tablespoons fat-free plain yogurt

2 tablespoons orange juice

1 1/2 teaspoons balsamic vinegar

3/4 teaspoon chopped fresh ginger

1/2 teaspoon grated orange peel

1/2 teaspoon Dijon mustard

2 tablespoons olive oil

1/4 teaspoon salt

1/8 teaspoon ground black pepper

6 cups fresh spinach, washed and dried

12 slices peeled cucumber (optional)

12 cherry or grape tomatoes (optional)

6 thinly sliced rings of red onion (optional)

In a small bowl, whisk together the yogurt, orange juice, vinegar, ginger, orange peel, and mustard. Gradually whisk in the oil. Season with the salt and pepper.

Toss the spinach with the dressing. Serve garnished with the cucumber, tomatoes, and onion, if using.

Makes 4 servings

Per serving: 87 calories, 3 g protein, 5 g carbohydrates, 7 g total fat, 1 g saturated fat, 0 mg cholesterol, 2 g dietary fiber, 208 mg sodium

ENTRÉES

Shrimp with Chard and Red Beans

Don't shy away from shrimp when you can make them a healthy part of your diet with a vegetable-packed meal like this!

4 cloves garlic, minced

1 1/2 teaspoons paprika

1 teaspoon dried thyme, crushed

½ teaspoon freshly ground black pepper
¼ teaspoon salt
¼ teaspoon ground red pepper
1 pound large shrimp, peeled and deveined, tails left on
2 tablespoons olive oil
2 ribs celery, thinly sliced
1 large onion, chopped
1 large green bell pepper, chopped
¾ cup chicken broth
3 cups green or red Swiss chard, thinly sliced
1 can (14–19 ounces) red kidney beans

In a medium bowl, combine the garlic, paprika, thyme, black pepper, salt, and red pepper. Remove about half of the mixture to a small bowl. Add the shrimp to the medium bowl and toss to coat well.

Heat 1 tablespoon of the oil in a large saucepot or Dutch oven over medium heat. Add the celery, onion, and bell pepper. Cook, stirring frequently, for 6 minutes, or until crisp-tender.

Add the reserved spice mixture and cook, stirring frequently, for 2 minutes. Add ¼ cup of the broth. Cover and cook, stirring often, for 5 minutes.

Add the chard and cook, stirring frequently, for 2 minutes, or until wilted. Stir in the beans, shrimp, and the remaining ½ cup broth and bring to a boil over high heat. Reduce the heat to low, cover, and simmer for 4 minutes, or until the shrimp are opaque.

Makes 4 servings
Per serving: 306 calories, 31 g protein, 26 g carbohydrates, 9 g total fat, 1 g saturated fat, 172 mg cholesterol, 9 g dietary fiber, 733 mg sodium

Mini-Salmon Cakes
The salmon in these fish cakes contains the heart disease–fighting power of omega-3 fatty acids. If you

prepare and form the cakes in the morning—or even
the day before—all they need is a light dip in crumbs
before cooking.

2 large eggs
4 teaspoons grated onion
1 tablespoon Dijon mustard
1 teaspoon Worcestershire sauce
¼ teaspoon salt
⅛ teaspoon ground black pepper
3 tablespoons finely chopped red bell pepper
2 teaspoons + 2 tablespoons ground flaxseed
4 teaspoons chopped fresh dill
1½ cup cooked, coarsely flaked salmon (canned or from 1
pound raw fillet)
4 teaspoons + 2 tablespoons dried bread crumbs
Lemon wedges

If you are starting with raw salmon, broil it 4" from the heat
for 3 minutes per side, or until it's opaque in the center.

In a large bowl, stir together the eggs, onion, mustard,
Worcestershire, salt, and black pepper until smooth. Stir in the
bell pepper, 2 teaspoons of the flaxseed, and dill. Fold in the
salmon and 4 teaspoons of the bread crumbs. Combine well.

Form the mixture into eight ½"-thick cakes. (They can be
refrigerated for up to 24 hours at this point.)

Mix together the remaining 2 tablespoons flaxseed and 2
tablespoons bread crumbs on a large plate. Coat the cakes on
all sides with the breading.

Coat a large, nonstick skillet with cooking spray, and set it
over low heat. When it's hot, add the cakes. Slowly brown
them on one side for 5 to 6 minutes. Turn them over, cover,
and cook until they are golden brown on the second side and
hot throughout, about 5 minutes. Serve with the lemon wedges.
Makes 8 cakes

Per 2-cake serving: 206 calories, 17 g protein, 11 g carbohydrates, 10 g total fat, 2 g saturated fat, 142 mg cholesterol, 3 g
dietary fiber, 632 mg sodium

Penne with Salmon and Roasted Vegetables
Mediterranean-inspired ingredients add color and flavor
to this special fish dish.

12 ounces penne
2 pounds leeks
1 red bell pepper, cut into strips
¼ cup chicken broth
2 tablespoons lemon juice
1 tablespoon olive oil
2 teaspoons dried thyme, crushed
¼ teaspoon freshly ground black pepper
1 yellow summer squash, halved and cut into ¼" slices
¼ cup pitted kalamata olives
1 salmon fillet (½ pound), skinned

Preheat the oven to 400°F. Prepare the pasta according to
package directions.

Meanwhile, cut the leeks into 2" lengths and quarter them
lengthwise. Rinse the leeks completely. Place the leeks and bell
pepper in a 13" x 9" baking dish. Add the broth, lemon juice, 2
teaspoons of the oil, thyme, and black pepper. Cover with foil
and bake for 15 minutes.

Add the squash, olives, and salmon to the baking dish and
drizzle with the remaining 1 teaspoon oil. Cover and bake for
30 minutes, or until the salmon is opaque and the vegetables
are tender.

Place the penne in a large serving bowl. Break the salmon
into bite-size pieces and add to the penne with the vegetables.
Makes 6 servings
Per serving: 402 calories, 18 g protein, 68 g carbohydrates, 7 g

total fat, 1 g saturated fat, 21 mg cholesterol, 5 g dietary fiber,
121 mg sodium

BBQ Butterflied Leg of Lamb
You will love this unique method of preparing delicious
lamb.
¼ cup extra-virgin olive oil
⅓ cup lemon juice
10 cloves garlic, minced
2 tablespoons chopped fresh rosemary or 2 teaspoons dried,
crushed
1 tablespoon grated lemon peel
1¼ teaspoons salt
1¼ teaspoons freshly ground black pepper
1 butterflied, well-trimmed leg of lamb (4 pounds)

In a large shallow baking dish or a large bowl, combine the oil,
lemon juice, garlic, rosemary, lemon peel, salt, and pepper.

Add the lamb and turn to coat well. Cover and refrigerate,
turning the lamb several times, overnight or for at least 2 hours.

Preheat a grill. Place the lamb on the grill rack and drizzle
with any remaining marinade. Grill, turning 2 or 3 times, for 25
to 35 minutes, or until a thermometer inserted in the thickest
part registers 145°F for medium-rare. (Thinner parts will be
more well-done.)

Place the lamb on a cutting board and let stand for 10
minutes. Cut into thin slices.
Makes 16 servings
*Per serving: 180 calories, 23 g protein, 1 g carbohydrates, 9 g
total fat, 2 g saturated fat, 73 mg cholesterol, 0 g dietary fiber,
253 mg sodium*

Pork Tenderloin with Vegetables
Presteaming the vegetables helps speed the cooking
time of this wonderful meal.

I pound small red potatoes, cut into 1"-thick wedges
3 large carrots, cut into 1" chunks
I tablespoon grated lemon peel
2 teaspoons dried rosemary, crushed, + rosemary sprigs for garnish
I teaspoon fennel seeds, crushed
¾ teaspoon cracked black pepper
½ teaspoon salt
I pound pork tenderloin
I teaspoon + I tablespoon extra-virgin olive oil
4 medium plum tomatoes, each cut into 4 wedges
I onion, cut into ½"-thick wedges
⅓ cup chicken broth

Preheat the oven to 450°F. Coat a roasting pan with cooking spray.

Place a steamer basket in a large saucepan with ½" of water. Place the potatoes and carrots in the steamer. Bring to a boil over high heat. Reduce the heat to medium, cover, and cook for 5 minutes, or until the potatoes are just tender. Remove from the heat.

Meanwhile, in a large bowl, combine the lemon peel, dried rosemary, fennel, pepper, and salt. Rub the pork with 2 teaspoons of the herb mixture. Place the pork in the center of the prepared roasting pan and drizzle with I teaspoon of the oil.

Add the potatoes and carrots, tomatoes, and onion to the herb mixture remaining in the bowl. Add the remaining I tablespoon oil and toss to coat well. Arrange the vegetables around the roast. Drizzle the vegetables with the broth.

Roast for 30 minutes, or until a thermometer inserted in the center reaches 155°F, the juices run clear, and the vegetables are tender and lightly browned on the edges. Place the pork on a cutting board and let stand for 5 minutes.

Slice the pork on the diagonal and place on a platter with the vegetables. Drizzle with the pan juices and garnish with rosemary sprigs.

Makes 4 servings

Per serving: 320 calories, 29 g protein, 31 g carbohydrates, 9 g total fat, 2 g saturated fat, 74 mg cholesterol, 6 g dietary fiber, 427 mg sodium

Chicken Piccata with Escarole

This traditional chicken dish features a delicious lemon-butter sauce.

4 boneless, skinless chicken breast halves
1/2 teaspoon dried thyme, crushed
1/4 teaspoon freshly ground black pepper
1/4 teaspoon salt
2 cloves garlic, minced
5 cups loosely packed cut-up escarole
1 cup cherry tomatoes, halved
1/2 cup fat-free chicken broth
2 teaspoons cornstarch
1/2 teaspoon grated lemon peel
1 tablespoon lemon juice
1 tablespoon butter

Coat the broiler-pan rack with cooking spray. Preheat the broiler.

Season both sides of the chicken breasts with the thyme, pepper, and 1/8 teaspoon of the salt. Place the chicken on the broiler-pan rack and broil 2" to 3" from the heat for 5 minutes per side, or until a thermometer inserted in the thickest portion registers 160°F and the juices run clear. Place the chicken on a platter and keep warm.

Meanwhile, heat a large skillet coated with cooking spray over medium-high heat. Add the garlic and cook, stirring constantly, for 30 seconds, or until fragrant. Add the escarole and cook, stirring frequently, for 3 minutes, or until the greens begin to wilt. Add the tomatoes and the remaining ⅛ teaspoon salt and cook for 3 minutes, or until the tomatoes are soft and the escarole is completely wilted. Place the vegetables on the platter with the chicken.

In a cup, combine the broth and cornstarch and stir until dissolved. In the same skillet, whisk together the cornstarch mixture, lemon peel, and lemon juice and bring to a boil over high heat, stirring constantly. Cook, stirring, for 1 minute, or until the sauce is slightly thickened. Add the butter and any juices that have collected on the platter and return to a boil, stirring constantly. Cook just until the butter is melted and the sauce has thickened. Pour the sauce over the chicken and vegetables.

Makes 4 servings

Per serving: 151 calories, 21 g protein, 6 g carbohydrates, 4 g total fat, 2 g saturated fat, 58 mg cholesterol, 3 g dietary fiber, 257 mg sodium

Jerk Chicken with Mango

Add excitement to any meal with this zesty chicken breast recipe.

2 jalapeño chile peppers, halved and seeded (wear plastic gloves when handling)

½ small onion, halved

2 cloves garlic, minced

1 slice (¼" thick) peeled fresh ginger

1 tablespoon olive oil

1 tablespoon white wine vinegar

1½ teaspoons dried thyme, crushed

1 teaspoon ground allspice

¼ teaspoon salt

4 skinless bone-in chicken breast halves

1 mango, peeled and diced
1 tablespoon chopped fresh mint

Preheat the oven to 450°F. Coat a 13" x 9" baking pan with cooking spray.

In a food processor, combine the peppers, onion, garlic, ginger, oil, vinegar, thyme, allspice, and salt. Process until very finely chopped, stopping the machine a few times to scrape down the sides of the container.

Spread the jalapeño mixture on both sides of the chicken breasts. Place them, skinned side up, in the prepared baking pan.

Bake for 30 minutes, or until a thermometer inserted in the thickest portion registers 170°F and the juices run clear.

Place the chicken on plates and scatter the mango on top. Sprinkle with the mint.

Makes 4 servings
Per serving: 199 calories, 26 g protein, 12 g carbohydrates, 5 g total fat, 1 g saturated fat, 64 mg cholesterol, 2 g dietary fiber, 220 mg sodium

Turkey and Bean Soft Tacos

A creamy cabbage and carrot filling makes a pleasing addition to this taco rendition.

8 corn tortillas (6" diameter)
8 ounces (2 cups) shredded cooked turkey breast
1 cup drained and rinsed canned kidney or pinto beans
1¼ cups mild or medium-spicy salsa + additional for topping
½ teaspoon ground cumin
1½ cups finely shredded cabbage
1 large carrot, shredded
¼ cup finely chopped sweet white onion
¼ cup reduced-fat cucumber ranch dressing

Preheat the oven to 350°F.

Stack the tortillas and wrap them in foil. Place the tortillas in the oven and heat for 10 minutes.

Meanwhile, heat a large skillet coated with cooking spray over high heat. Add the turkey, beans, 1¼ cups of the salsa, and cumin and bring to a boil. Reduce the heat to low, cover, and simmer, stirring, for 10 minutes, or until heated through.

In a medium bowl, combine the cabbage, carrot, onion, and ranch dressing.

Spoon about ⅓ cup of the turkey filling into a tortilla. Top with ¼ cup of the cabbage mixture and fold over. Repeat with the remaining tortillas, turkey filling, and cabbage mixture. Top with the remaining salsa.

Makes 4 servings

Per serving: 330 calories, 24 g protein, 44 g carbohydrates, 6 g total fat, 1 g saturated fat, 47 mg cholesterol, 8 g dietary fiber, 676 mg sodium

One-Pot Chicken and Rice

This convenient meal calls for pantry staples like canned tomatoes and brown rice, and really only requires one ovenproof pot from beginning to end.

2 tablespoons olive oil

3 cloves garlic, minced

1 large onion, chopped

1¼ cups brown rice

4 chicken thighs, skin and visible fat removed

1 can (14½ ounces) diced tomatoes, drained

2 cups chicken broth

1 teaspoon dried thyme, crushed

½ teaspoon freshly ground black pepper

Preheat the oven to 325°F.

Heat the oil in an ovenproof Dutch oven over medium heat.

Add the garlic and onion and cook, stirring frequently, for 4 minutes, or until softened.

Add the rice and cook, stirring, for 2 minutes, or until it starts to brown. Stir in the chicken, tomatoes, broth, thyme, and pepper. Bring to a boil over high heat.

Cover the pot and place in the oven. Bake for 1 hour and 15 minutes, or until the rice is tender and the liquid is absorbed.

Makes 4 servings

Per serving: 392 calories, 20 g protein, 52 g carbohydrates, 11 g total fat, 2 g saturated fat, 57 mg cholesterol, 4 g dietary fiber, 537 mg sodium

DESSERTS

Creamy Chocolate Cheesecake

This amazing cheesecake uses less butter than most recipes, along with reduced-fat cream cheese for a divine chocolate treat.

18 chocolate graham crackers

2 tablespoons butter or trans-free margarine, melted

3 packages (8 ounces each) reduced-fat cream cheese, softened

1½ cups sugar

1 egg

2 egg whites

¾ cups cocoa powder

¼ teaspoon salt

1 tablespoon vanilla extract

½ teaspoon almond extract

½ cup fat-free whipped topping

½ cup raspberries

1 cup fat-free caramel sauce, warmed

Preheat the oven to 325°F. Coat a 9" springform pan with cooking spray.

Place the graham crackers in a plastic food-storage bag. Seal, then crush with a rolling pin until the crackers form coarse crumbs. Place in the prepared pan with the butter. Stir to combine, and press the crumb mixture onto the bottom and up the side of the pan. Bake for 10 minutes, or until set. Remove to a rack to cool.

In a large bowl, with an electric mixer at medium speed, beat the cream cheese and sugar until smooth. Add the egg, egg whites, cocoa, salt, vanilla extract, and almond extract. Beat for 5 minutes, or until smooth and well-combined. Pour into the prepared crust. Bake for 1¼ hours, or until the center is slightly soft. Turn off the oven, and leave the cake in the oven for 1 hour. Remove to a rack and cool for 1 hour. Cover and refrigerate for 2 hours or overnight.

Serve with whipped topping, raspberries, and warmed caramel sauce.

Makes 16 servings

Per serving: 272 calories, 7 g protein, 35 g carbohydrates, 11 g total fat, 6 g saturated fat, 41 mg cholesterol, 2 g dietary fiber, 275 mg sodium

Apple Crumble with Toasted-Oat Topping

Try this guilt-free apple dessert when you are craving apple pie!

6 medium Jonagold or Golden Delicious apples, cored and thinly sliced
½ cup unsweetened applesauce
¾ cup rolled oats
3 tablespoons toasted wheat germ
3 tablespoons packed light brown sugar
1 teaspoon ground cinnamon
1 tablespoon canola oil
1 tablespoon unsalted butter, cut into small pieces

Preheat the oven to 350°F. Coat a 13" x 9" baking dish with cooking spray.

Combine the apples and applesauce in the prepared baking dish.

In a small bowl, combine the oats, wheat germ, brown sugar, and cinnamon. Add the oil and butter. Mix with your fingers to form crumbs. Sprinkle the oat mixture evenly over the apples.

Bake for 30 minutes, or until the topping is golden and the apples are bubbling.

Makes 6 servings

Per serving: 207 calories, 3 g protein, 38 g carbohydrates, 6 g total fat, 2 g saturated fat, 5 mg cholesterol, 6 g dietary fiber, 3 mg sodium

Creamy Mousse with Concord Grape Sauce

This simple mousse is a good source of calcium and a wonderful way to add heart-healthy nuts to your diet.

1 cup reduced-fat ricotta cheese
⅔ cup fat-free plain yogurt
7 tablespoons confectioners' sugar, sifted
½ teaspoon grated lemon peel
½ teaspoon vanilla extract
¼ teaspoon ground cinnamon
1 teaspoon gelatin powder
2 tablespoons cold water
⅓ cup Concord grape juice
¾ teaspoon cornstarch
¼ cup toasted pecans, chopped

In a medium bowl, mix together the ricotta, yogurt, sugar, lemon peel, vanilla extract, and cinnamon.

Sprinkle the gelatin over the water in a small saucepan and let it soften for 1 minute. Set the saucepan over very low heat and dissolve the gelatin, stirring for 1 minute. Let it cool.

Stir the gelatin into the ricotta mixture thoroughly. Transfer to a serving bowl or 4 stemmed glasses. Refrigerate until it has set, 2 to 3 hours or overnight.

Measure 1 tablespoon of the juice into a small bowl and mix in the cornstarch.

Bring the remaining juice to a low boil in a small saucepan. Whisk in the cornstarch mixture. Boil the sauce, whisking, until it becomes shiny, clear, and thickened, about 1 minute. Let the sauce cool (or refrigerate it for up to 3 days).

Drizzle each serving with the sauce and sprinkle with the pecans.

Makes 4 servings

Per serving: 215 calories, 10 g protein, 21 g carbohydrates, 10 g total fat, 3 g saturated fat, 20 mg cholesterol, 0.5 g dietary fiber, 107 mg sodium

Ginger Pumpkin Pie

This pie features a delicious whole wheat crust that helps make this wholesome pumpkin dessert even healthier.

1 1/4 cups whole wheat pastry flour
1/4 teaspoon + 1/8 teaspoon salt
3 tablespoons canola oil
2 tablespoons cold butter, cut into small pieces
2–4 tablespoons ice water
1/2 cup packed brown sugar
1 egg
2 egg whites
1 1/2 teaspoons vanilla extract
1/2 teaspoon ground cinnamon
1/2 teaspoon ground ginger
1/4 teaspoon ground nutmeg

1 can (15 ounces) plain pumpkin
1 cup fat-free evaporated milk

In a food processor, combine the flour and ¼ teaspoon of the salt. Pulse until blended. Add the oil and butter. Pulse until the mixture resembles a fine meal. Add the water, 1 tablespoon at a time, as needed, and pulse just until the dough forms large clumps. Form into a ball and flatten into a disk. Cover and refrigerate for at least 1 hour.

Preheat the oven to 425°F. Coat a 9" pie plate with cooking spray.

Place the dough between 2 pieces of waxed paper and roll into a 12" circle. Remove the top piece of paper and invert the dough into the pie plate. Peel off the second piece of paper. Press the dough into the pie plate and up onto the rim, patching where necessary. Turn under the rim and flute. Chill in the refrigerator.

Meanwhile, in a large bowl, whisk the brown sugar, egg, egg whites, vanilla extract, cinnamon, ginger, nutmeg, and the remaining ⅛ teaspoon salt until well-blended. Whisk in the pumpkin and milk. Pour into the chilled crust. Bake for 15 minutes. Reduce the temperature to 350°F. Bake for 25 minutes, or until a knife inserted off-center comes out clean. Cool on a rack.

Makes 8 servings
Per serving: 252 calories, 7 g protein, 36 g carbohydrates, 9 g total fat, 3 g saturated fat, 36 mg cholesterol, 4 g dietary fiber, 217 mg sodium

PART V

Success Stories

Making improvements in your life can be a daunting experience, even when you know that the changes will bring you better health.

But sometimes starting with just one change can trigger a domino effect that sets off improvements across many areas of your life. That was the case with the people who share their cholesterol success stories in the following five chapters.

Take a look at the obstacles they overcame and the creativity they used to bring their cholesterol down to a heart-healthy level, then put their Take-Home Message to work in your own life.

CHAPTER FOURTEEN

Now He Knows What He's Eating

Jim McDonnell's kids used to love when he grocery-shopped.

"All the junk they wanted to eat, I would buy for them," says Jim, 69, a retired insurance sales manager from Salisbury Township, Pennsylvania. "Now, I don't put anything in the basket without reading the label. I have learned to eat smart."

In 1997, Jim's cholesterol hovered around 300. But he was not worried about it, until he started experiencing muscle weakness in his legs caused by an arterial blockage. In early 2000, he had his right carotid artery operated on to clean out plaque buildup. "It was even more serious than the testing had indicated," he says.

After the surgery, his doctor recommended that he participate in a cholesterol-reduction study taking place at Lehigh Valley Hospital in Allentown. It's called LOVAR (Lowering of Vascular Atherosclerotic Risk) and combines nutrition and exercise classes with medication. Jim takes pravastatin (Pravachol), Plavix (an aspirin substitute), a multivitamin, and supplements of vitamins C and E, folic acid, calcium, magnesium, and zinc.

Following the advice of a physical therapist, he has built up to 30 minutes a day on the treadmill. When he started, he could go only 2 minutes on it before having to rest.

After 4 months of nutrition classes, he cut way back on red meat. He replaced high-fat ice cream with fat-free frozen yogurt, increased his vegetable and fruit intake to nine servings a day, and learned to check out the fat content and ingredients of products before buying them. "Before, I never gave that one iota of thought," he says. "I was a lazy eater. Anything I could put in my mouth, I put in."

At his most recent screening, his cholesterol was 230—still too high, he says. He wants to get to 200. On the plus side, he has lost 10 pounds. He's 5 feet 11, and he did weigh 190. Now he's only 5 pounds from his goal of 175.

"I used to think nothing about a couple of doughnuts for breakfast," Jim says. "I didn't really know what was in them, nutritionwise. Now I know." These days, breakfast is a bowl of bran cereal or oatmeal with a soy–cow's milk blend.

Lunch, at one time a cheeseburger or a sandwich "with any kind of meat," is now a tuna sandwich with light mayonnaise. Steak for dinner has been replaced with lean meat and vegetables flavored with a cholesterol-lowering margarine.

"I used to be a big snacker," he adds. "I don't snack anymore."

Jim says that he feels great. He is happy to be able to enjoy trips to New York City and Europe with his wife, Bunny.

"Hardly a week goes by that I don't hear of a friend having a health problem," he says. "Maybe it is because of their lifestyles. They are doing the very thing I was doing: too much of what's not good for you."

TAKE-HOME MESSAGE

Understand what you're putting in your mouth. Too many tasty and easy-to-eat foods—packaged cookies, doughnuts, potato chips, fast-food cheeseburgers—are loaded with fat. And "low-cholesterol" or "no-cholesterol" claims don't mean that the foods can't be loaded with hydrogenated oils, which may be no better for you than animal fats. Your first step toward eating better is understanding how food ingredients affect your cholesterol. The second step is making sure the undesirable ingredients are not hidden in the snacks you love. As always, diligent label reading is essential. When you really understand that something is not good for you, the temptation to eat it fades.

CHAPTER FIFTEEN

She Replaced High-Fat Favorites with Low-Fat Versions

On most days for lunch, Jessie Maurer used to eat a double cheeseburger with bacon and two large orders of fries at a fast-food restaurant. But when her cholesterol hit 299 in 1998, Jessie quickly learned the art of substitution, replacing all her high-fat favorites with low-fat alternatives.

Cheeseburgers became burgers made of portobello mushrooms or ground turkey. Omelettes were prepared with egg substitute. French fries were ditched in favor of baked potato wedges seasoned with olive oil and herbs. "I realized I could eat a lot of things," says Jessie, 54, of Emmaus, Pennsylvania. "I just had to eat them a different way."

Although she walks ¾ mile to work every day, Jessie had a weight problem for years. But she never gave much thought to her cholesterol levels until she went through menopause in 1998 and her doctor suggested she have them checked out. "When he saw my results, he told me I was a ticking time bomb," she recalls.

"My doctor, who had had heart surgery himself, told me to cut out the fat. If changing my diet didn't work, he was going to put me on medications."

Eager to avoid taking drugs, Jessie went on a quest for low-fat substitutes. She was surprised to discover that it was easier than crash dieting, which for Jessie had always meant a week of eating nothing but plain tuna. "I had crash-dieted so many times and always felt deprived," she says. "This was so much easier because I wasn't really depriving myself; I was just eating in a different way."

Initially, the hardest part was grocery shopping. "Before, I never looked at labels, and I'd just throw things in the cart," she says. "Now, I had to pull my glasses out and read everything." What was once a 20-minute trip to the supermarket turned into an hour, as she learned to read nutrition labels and weed out the foods high in fat, cholesterol, and saturated fat.

Her vigilance has paid off in a lower cholesterol level, which fell to 210 by December 2000. She has also lost more than 60 pounds, dropping from a high of 186 in 1998 to her current weight of 124 on her 5-foot-7 frame.

The only food she could not adequately replace was mayonnaise, which has meant giving up two of her old favorites: macaroni and potato salads. "That was hard at first," says Jessie, who used to make a big bowl of one or the other and eat it through the week. "Pasta salads with low-fat dressing just aren't the same. So every once in a while, I'll sneak a little taste."

TAKE-HOME MESSAGE

Replace your high-fat faves with lower-fat ones. Low-fat substitutes for cholesterol-raising foods are abundant. Use them! If you make chili with ground turkey instead of ground beef, you eat 27 percent less fat. If you substitute frozen chocolate yogurt for chocolate ice cream, you save another 45 percent fat. Peruse magazines, cookbooks, and the Internet for low-fat recipes of your favorite dishes. By making healthier versions of high-fat foods instead of banning them from your diet, you'll be less likely to feel deprived and more likely to stick with good eating habits.

CHAPTER SIXTEEN

He Made a Fast Break
from Fast Food

In his job as a recreation and sports director, Glen Flood works closely with nutrition, heart, stroke, and diabetes organizations to promote active living and an awareness of healthy lifestyles.

But until recently, the 30-year-old found it much easier to talk the talk than to walk the walk. "I used to believe that if I exercised some, I'd be okay to eat fast food," says Glen, who lives in Charlottetown, Prince Edward Island. "I'd think I was hungry, snack way too much between meals, and eat a lot of burgers and fries as well as deep-fried foods."

The "snack now, work out later" policy didn't fare well. "Exercise was way too often put on the back burner," says Glen. "I'd put it off until the next day because I was convinced that I could get fit later."

Glen didn't pay much attention to his health until he and his fiancée started attending seminars sponsored by a company that markets supplements. "The seminars had stats about people as young as I am having serious illness caused by high cholesterol," he says. "They also presented everyone with pamphlets that had information about heredity and how high cholesterol runs in families.

"I have a family history of high blood pressure, high cholesterol, and heart problems," Glen continues. In the winter of 1998, he found out that his total cholesterol reading was over 300, and his LDL level was 208. "That was a good reason to start making life changes," he says.

Even with the same busy work schedule, Glen says he now packs his lunch instead of heading for his favorite fast-food haunts. "I do my best not to snack," he says, "and when I do snack, I make it apples, oranges, and other fruit."

Glen has also made a point of committing himself to regular exercise. Drawing on his experience as a recreation director, he has tried out various activities, from circuit training to basketball to soccer. "Over time," he says, "exercise has become fun again, and I no longer see it as a task."

Since 1999, Glen has lowered his total cholesterol to a much healthier 200 and his LDL to 134. He's also lost 20 pounds, bringing himself down to a trimmer 160 pounds on his 5-foot-6 frame. "My awareness and knowledge have improved 100 percent," says Glen. "The changes have not been easy, but they've been positive!"

TAKE-HOME MESSAGE

Kick the fast-food habit. You probably realize that fast food isn't good for you, but do you really know what you're getting at the takeout window? A quarter-pound burger with cheese and super-size fries from McDonald's, for example, contain 59 grams of fat (18 grams of which are saturated). That's 90 percent of the total fat and saturated fat you should have in a day. One slice of a cheese stuffed-crust pizza from Pizza Hut contains 10 grams of saturated fat—half the daily recommended amount.

If your workplace doesn't have a cafeteria, bring a bagged lunch instead of going out to eat. And when you drive around town, carry fruit in the car so you can avoid the drive-thrus.

CHAPTER SEVENTEEN

He Bulked Up with Fiber—and Beat Cholesterol Cold

Terry Terfinko wasn't feeling his usual self. The Emmaus, Pennsylvania, resident didn't have as much energy as he used to, and he didn't feel as mentally sharp. Not only that, but he was worried because his mother's side of the family had heart and cholesterol problems. So he went for a checkup.

At the doctor's office, Terry's fears were realized: His cholesterol was 213 and his triglycerides were 346. At 234 pounds, he was 50 pounds over his high school weight. And to top it all off, he had high blood pressure.

Terry knew that he had to change his habits; his days of eating greasy cheesesteaks and fries were over. He read up on nutrition and learned that eating high-fiber meals would keep him fuller longer so that he could eat less and still not feel deprived. "I started eating more fruits and vegetables. And I came to like seven-grain cereals," Terry says. "I make a mix of psyllium and oat bran and sprinkle it on cereal. I even put it in bread and pancakes. Eating more fiber makes my stomach feel full."

Switching to high-fiber foods wasn't hard for Terry. It was just a matter of making some clever substitutions, such as whole wheat bread for white and high-fiber cereal in place of regular. And he didn't even miss the high-fat, high-calorie foods he cut out. "When I eat those old foods now, it doesn't feel good," he says. "It got so that I came to prefer foods in their natural state—a potato instead of french fries or potato chips, whole fresh fruit instead of canned."

Besides going the high-fiber route, Terry became a biking devotee, increasing his endurance until he was cycling more than 5,000 miles per year.

It worked. Two years after his initial diagnosis, Terry learned that his cholesterol was down to 143 and his triglycerides had dropped to 90. "My doctor was amazed at the results," he says. "I went off the blood pressure meds. My weight is currently 182 pounds, and at age 48, I have the energy of a 20-year-old."

TAKE-HOME MESSAGE

Reach for high-fiber foods. Make it your mission to find sneaky but simple ways to get more fiber into your diet. You'll feel full while eating less food. And the fiber itself can actually help lower your cholesterol. Read labels carefully so that you can replace low-fiber breads and cereals with their high-fiber counterparts. Sprinkle wheat germ, psyllium, and oat bran on cereal, yogurt, and ice cream. Or use them to replace some of the flour in homemade pancakes and bread.

CHAPTER EIGHTEEN

He Beat Cholesterol One Step at a Time

In the old days, Ernest Laabs finished off a good meal by plopping down on the couch in front of the television. These days, he's more apt to take a 15-minute walk after every one of his meals. "The object is to get the body moving and circulating, just to get all this stuff moving," says the 69-year-old San Bernardino, California, resident.

Ernest had a massive heart attack in 1991, and his cholesterol hit 350. "The doctors told me that if I behaved, I could live maybe another 5 years," Ernest recalls. Five years later, he was diagnosed with diabetes.

By the summer of 2000, Ernest was taking 27 pills a day to control his myriad ailments, which by then included high blood pressure. He also had a calcified artery in his leg, which kept him up nights, pacing in pain. An outspoken friend of his wife, Elayne, took a look at him one day and asked her if she was prepared to spend the rest of her life alone. That was all Elayne needed to drag her husband to the NewStart Lifestyle Program in Weimar, California, a facility that helps patients improve their health through diet and exercise. "I was not pleased with the idea of going," Ernest says. "I said, 'This has got to be a joke.' But I went because I promised I'd love, honor, and obey her."

After 18 days at the NewStart program, Ernest returned home a changed person. He eliminated steak, his favorite food, from his diet altogether. He also gave up cheese, eggs, and butter, and switched from regular milk to soy milk. Now he builds his meals around tofu, homemade grain breads, and fresh fruits and vegetables.

He also learned to take a 15-minute walk after every meal. Sometimes, he simply paces his 2,000-square-foot house or goes up and down the stairs. Other times, he walks around the yard or circles the neighborhood. "You don't need a park to walk," Ernest says. "You just have to get out there and do it."

Improvements in his diet and exercise have made it easier for Ernest to enjoy his favorite activity: square dancing. "It used to tucker me out like you wouldn't believe," he says. "If I danced for 15 minutes straight, it was great. Now, I could dance all evening. On New Year's Eve, I danced from 7:30 to 12:30. I didn't want to quit, but everybody else did."

He also cut the number of pills he takes to just three a day—none of which are for his cholesterol, which dropped most recently to 155. His leg no longer bothers him at all, and he shed 16 pounds in the 6 months after he went to the NewStart program. At 5 feet 10 inches, he now weighs 164 pounds.

TAKE-HOME MESSAGE

Take a short walk after every meal. Rather than slump in front of the TV after dinner, commit yourself to doing some activity, be it a short walk in the house or a longer one outdoors. By moving immediately after eating, you'll sneak in some extra exercise. And for those with diabetes, the exercise helps stabilize blood sugars. If lying on the couch is your habit, ask your spouse or a friend to encourage you, even join you. Ask someone else to hide the remote control. Get dressed for your walk before dinner or tape a big reminder note onto the refrigerator. The goal is to create a new habit of exercise.

FAT AND
CHOLESTEROL COUNTER

Like most other fat and cholesterol counters, this chart divvies up foods to categories. Since beans, grains, fruits, and vegetables typically contain little or no saturated fat and cholesterol, we've decided to devote the most space to foods that sometimes cause people problems. What you'll find are common categories from breakfast foods to salad dressings. In between, you'll find desserts, fish and shellfish, meats, and many more.

But this chart is designed a bit differently from those you may have used in the past. It ranks foods by the amount of saturated fat per serving, from highest to lowest in each category. Most experts agree that saturated fat is the healthy heart's worst enemy. The less saturated fat you eat, the healthier your diet will be—as long as your overall calorie and cholesterol intakes are reasonable, that is. As odd as it may seem, some foods contain a low percentage of saturated fat but pack lots of calories and cholesterol. For example, a couple of slices of frozen French toast drizzled with low-calorie syrup will "cost" you less than 2 grams of saturated fat, but in exchange, they provide significant calories and cholesterol.

We've rounded calorie and cholesterol counts to the

nearest whole number and fat and saturated fat values to the nearest tenth of a gram. Foods that get less than 1 percent of their calories per serving from fat or saturated fat are designated by "1."

FOOD	PORTION	CALORIES	FAT (G)
BREAKFAST FOODS			
Croissant with egg, cheese, and sausage (Burger King)	1 (about 6 oz)	530	41
Croissant with ham and cheese (Arby's)	1 (about 4¼ oz)	345	20.7
Biscuit with egg and sausage (McDonald's)	1 (about 6½ oz)	520	35
Croissant	1 (about 2 oz)	235	12
Pancakes with 2 pats butter and syrup (McDonald's)	3 (about 9 oz total)	560	14
French toast, frozen, with low-calorie syrup	2 slices (about 4 oz total) with 4 Tbsp syrup	340	6
Bran muffin, homemade with wheat bran and 2% milk	1 (about 2 oz)	161	7
Cinnamon roll, refrigerator, baked, with frosting	1 (about 1 oz)	109	4
Toaster pastry with fruit	1	204	5.3
Waffle, frozen, with low-calorie syrup	1 (about 1¼ oz) with 2 Tbsp syrup	136	2.1

SATURATED FAT (G)	% CALORIES FROM FAT	% CALORIES FROM SATURATED FAT	CHOLESTEROL (mg)
14	69.6	23.8	255
12.1	54	31.6	90
10	60.6	17.3	245
3.5	46	13.4	13
2.5	22.5	4	10
1.5	15.9	4	80
1.3	39.1	7.3	19
1	33	8.3	0
0.8	23.4	3.5	0
0.5	13.9	3.3	0

FOOD	PORTION	CALORIES	FAT (G)
Bagel, plain or onion	1 (about 2½ oz)	195	1.1

CHEESE

FOOD	PORTION	CALORIES	FAT (G)
Ricotta, regular	½ cup	216	16.1
Ricotta, reduced-fat	½ cup	171	9.8
Cheddar, regular	1 oz	110	9
Cream cheese, regular	1 oz	100	10
American	1 oz	106	8.9
Monterey Jack	1 oz	105	8.5
Blue cheese	1 oz	99	8.1
Mozzarella, regular	1 oz	79	6.1
Cream cheese, reduced-fat	2 Tbsp	70	5
Cheddar, reduced-fat	1 oz	80	5
Mozzarella, reduced-fat	1 oz	71	4.5
Parmesan, grated	1 Tbsp	23	1.5
Cottage cheese, 1%	½ cup	82	1.2
Cheddar, fat-free	1 oz	45	0

SATURATED FAT (G)	% CALORIES FROM FAT	% CALORIES FROM SATURATED FAT	CHOLESTEROL (mg)
0.2	5.1	1	0
10.3	67.1	42.9	63
6.1	51.6	32.1	38
6	73.6	49	30
6	90	54	30
5.6	75.6	47.5	27
5.3	72.9	45.4	25
5.2	73.6	47.3	21
3.7	69.5	42.2	22
3.5	64.3	45	15
3	56.3	33.8	20
2.8	57	35.5	16
1	58.7	39.1	4
0.7	13.2	7.7	5
0	0	0	25

FOOD	PORTION	CALORIES	FAT (G)
Cream cheese, fat-free	2 Tbsp	30	0

DESSERTS

Cakes and Cookies

FOOD	PORTION	CALORIES	FAT (G)
Cheesecake	¼ cake (about 4¼ oz)	350	18
Carrot cake, homemade with cream cheese icing	1 slice (¹⁄₁₂ of cake)	484	29.3
Devil's food, made from mix with eggs and oil, with 2 Tbsp chocolate icing	1 slice (¹⁄₁₂ of cake)	440	21
Sandwich, vanilla with cream filling	4 (about 2 oz total)	297	13.5
Fig bars	2 (about 1 oz total)	110	2.5
Brownie with nuts, made from mix	1 (about ¾ oz)	81	3.7
Oatmeal with raisins, homemade	1 (about ½ oz)	65	2.4
Angel food	1 slice (¹⁄₁₂ of cake)	73	0.2

Ice Cream and Frozen Treats

FOOD	PORTION	CALORIES	FAT (G)
Ice cream, vanilla, regular	½ cup	170	10

SATURATED FAT (G)	% CALORIES FROM FAT	% CALORIES FROM SATURATED FAT	CHOLESTEROL (mg)
0	0	0	5
9	46.3	23.1	50
5.4	54.5	10	60
4.5	43	9.2	45
3.7	41	11.2	23
1	20.5	8.2	0
0.6	41.1	6.6	13
0.5	33.2	6.9	5
0	2.5	1	0
6	52.9	31.8	105

FOOD	PORTION	CALORIES	FAT (G)
Ice cream, soft-serve, chocolate or vanilla, on cone	1 (about 5 oz)	230	7
Ice cream, vanilla, reduced-fat	½ cup	130	4.5
Ice milk, soft-serve, vanilla	½ cup	112	2.3
Sherbet, orange	½ cup	135	1.9
Frozen yogurt, vanilla, regular	½ cup	110	1.5
Ice cream, vanilla, low-fat	½ cup	100	2
Frozen yogurt, vanilla, fat-free	½ cup	110	0
Fruit ice	1 cup	247	0
Pies			
Apple, fresh	1 slice (⅛ of pie)	302	13.1
Pecan, fresh	1 slice (⅛ of pie)	431	23.6
Lemon meringue, fresh	1 slice (⅛ of pie)	268	10.7
Pudding and Gelatin			
Chocolate pudding, made from mix with whole milk	½ cup	163	4.6

SATURATED FAT (G)	% CALORIES FROM FAT	% CALORIES FROM SATURATED FAT	CHOLESTEROL (mg)
5	27.4	19.6	20
3	31.2	20.8	35
1.4	18.5	11.3	7
1.2	12.7	8	7
1	12.3	8.2	5
1	18	9	5
0	0	0	0
0	0	0	0
3.4	39	10.1	0
3.3	49.3	6.9	65
3.2	35.9	10.7	98
2.7	25.4	14.9	16

FOOD	PORTION	CALORIES	FAT (G)
Rice pudding with raisins, homemade	½ cup	194	4.1
Vanilla pudding, made from mix with 2% milk	½ cup	148	2.4
Gelatin, made from powder, with fruit	½ cup	80	0.1

Eggs and Egg Substitute

FOOD	PORTION	CALORIES	FAT (G)
Quiche Lorraine	1 slice (about 6 ¼ oz)	600	48
Egg, scrambled with butter and whole milk	1 large	95	7.1
Egg, fried with margarine	1 large	92	6.9
Egg yolk	1 large	59	5.1
Egg, hard-cooked	1 large	78	5.3
Egg substitute, liquid	¼ cup	53	2.1
Egg white	1 large	16	Trace

FAST FOODS

FOOD	PORTION	CALORIES	FAT (G)
Taco salad with small chili and 1 packet sour cream (Wendy's)	1 (about 30 oz)	830	42
Roast beef on bun (Arby's)	1 (about 6 oz)	383	18.2

SATURATED FAT (G)	% CALORIES FROM FAT	% CALORIES FROM SATURATED FAT	CHOLESTEROL (mg)
2.2	19	10.2	15
1.4	14.6	8.5	9
0	1.1	0	0
23.2	72	34.8	285
2.8	67.3	26.5	248
1.9	67.5	18.6	211
1.6	77.8	24.4	213
1.6	61.2	18.5	212
0.4	35.7	7	1
0	Trace	0	0
17.5	45.5	19	125
7	42.8	16.4	43

FOOD	PORTION	CALORIES	FAT (G)
Pizza, pepperoni (Domino's hand-tossed)	2 slices of 12" pie (about 6 oz)	406	15.1
Pizza, cheese (Domino's thin crust)	⅓ of 12" pie (about 5½ oz)	364	15.5
Pizza, sausage (Domino's hand-tossed)	2 slices of 12" pie with mushrooms (about 6 oz)	402	13.9
Cheeseburger with condiments on bun (Burger King)	1 (about 5 oz)	320	13
Hot dog, plain, on bun (Dairy Queen/Brazier)	1 (about 3 oz)	280	16
Nachos Supreme (Taco Bell)	1 order	364	18
Pizza, sausage (Pizza Hut)	1 slice of medium pie (about 4 oz)	267	11
Taco, beef (Taco Bell)	1	180	11
Baked potato with cheese and bacon (Wendy's)	1 (about 10 oz)	530	18
Baked potato with sour cream and chives (Wendy's)	1 (about 10 oz)	380	6

SATURATED FAT (G)	% CALORIES FROM FAT	% CALORIES FROM SATURATED FAT	CHOLESTEROL (mg)
6.6	33.8	14.6	32
6.3	38.3	15.6	26
6.1	31.1	13.7	31
6	36.6	16.9	40
6	51.4	19.3	25
5	44.5	12.4	17
5	37	16	31
5	55	25	32
4	30.6	6.8	20
4	14.2	9.5	15

FOOD	PORTION	CALORIES	FAT (G)
Burrito, bean (Taco Bell)	1	391	12
Chicken nuggets without sauce (KFC)	6 (about 3 oz total)	284	18
French fries (McDonald's)	1 large (about 6 oz)	450	22
Pizza, cheese (Pizza Hut thin crust)	1 slice of medium pie (about 3½ oz)	205	8
Chicken breast and wing quarter, roasted, without skin (KFC)	About 4 oz total	199	5.9
Fish, breaded, baked, without bun (Long John Silver's)	3 pieces (about 5 oz total)	150	1

FATS, OILS, AND SPREADS

Fats and Oils

FOOD	PORTION	CALORIES	FAT (G)
Coconut oil	1 Tbsp	120	13.6
Palm oil	1 Tbsp	120	13.6
Lard	1 Tbsp	115	12.8
Shortening	1 Tbsp	113	12.8
Soybean oil	1 Tbsp	120	13.6

SATURATED FAT (G)	% CALORIES FROM FAT	% CALORIES FROM SATURATED FAT	CHOLESTEROL (mg)
4	27.6	9.2	5
4	57	12.7	68
4	44	8	0
4	35.1	17.6	25
1.7	26.7	7.7	97
0.6	6	3.6	110
11.8	100	88.5	0
6.7	100	50.3	0
5	100	39.1	4
3.2	100	25.5	0
2	100	15	0

FOOD	PORTION	CALORIES	FAT (G)
Olive oil	1 Tbsp	119	13.5
Corn oil	1 Tbsp	120	13.6
Spreads			
Butter, salted or unsalted, stick or whipped	1 Tbsp	102	11.5
Peanut butter with added oils, smooth	2 Tbsp	188	16
Butter blend, made with butter and vegetable oil	1 Tbsp	50	6
Margarine, stick regular	1 Tbsp	100	11
Peanut butter without added oils	2 Tbsp	200	16
Margarine, squeeze	1 Tbsp	80	9
Mayonnaise, regular	1 Tbsp	100	11
Margarine, stick, reduced-fat	1 Tbsp	60	6
Margarine, tub, reduced-fat	1 Tbsp	45	4.5
Mayonnaise, reduced-fat	1 Tbsp	50	5
Mayonnaise, low-fat	1 Tbsp	25	1

SATURATED FAT (G)	% CALORIES FROM FAT	% CALORIES FROM SATURATED FAT	CHOLESTEROL (mg)
1.8	100	13.6	0
1.7	100	12.8	0
7.2	100	63.5	31
3.1	76.6	14.8	0
3	100	54	10
2	99	18	0
2	72	9	0
1.5	100	16.9	0
1.5	99	13.5	5
1	90	15	0
1	90	20	0
1	90	18	5
0	36	0	0

FOOD	PORTION	CALORIES	FAT (G)

FISH AND SHELLFISH

Fish

FOOD	PORTION	CALORIES	FAT (G)
Mackerel, Atlantic, broiled, baked, or microwaved	3 oz	223	15.1
Catfish, channel, breaded and fried	3 oz	195	11.3
Salmon, sockeye, fresh, broiled, baked, or microwaved	3 oz	184	9.3
Salmon pink, canned, with bones and liquid	3 oz	118	5.1
Trout, rainbow, broiled, baked, or microwaved	3 oz	128	3.7
Anchovies, canned in olive oil	5 (about ¾ oz total)	42	1.9
Bass, striped, uncooked	3 oz	82	2
Sardines, Atlantic, canned in oil, drained, with bones	2 (about 1 oz total)	50	2.8
Sole, broiled, baked, or microwaved	3 oz	99	1.3
Pollack, broiled, baked, or microwaved	3 oz	96	1

SATURATED FAT (G)	% CALORIES FROM FAT	% CALORIES FROM SATURATED FAT	CHOLESTEROL (mg)
3.6	60.9	14.5	64
2.8	52.2	12.9	69
1.6	45.5	7.8	74
1.3	38.9	9.9	47
0.7	26	4.9	62
0.4	40.7	8.6	17
0.4	22	4.4	68
0.4	50.4	7.2	34
0.3	11.8	2.7	58
0.2	9.4	1.9	82

FOOD	PORTION	CALORIES	FAT (G)
Tuna, light meat, canned in water	3 oz	99	0.7
Cod, Atlantic, broiled, baked, or microwaved	3 oz	89	0.7
Haddock, broiled, baked, or microwaved	3 oz	95	0.8
Shellfish			
Shrimp, mixed species, breaded and fried	3 oz	206	10.4
Scallops, mixed species, breaded and fried	2 large (about 1 oz total)	67	3.4
Shrimp, mixed species, steamed	3 oz	84	0.9
Clams, steamed	20 small (about 3 oz)	133	1.8
Crab, Alaskan king, steamed	3 oz	82	1.3
Lobster, boiled, poached, or steamed	3 oz	83	0.5
Scallops, uncooked	3 oz	75	0.7

SATURATED FAT (G)	% CALORIES FROM FAT	% CALORIES FROM SATURATED FAT	CHOLESTEROL (mg)
0.2	6.4	1.8	26
0.1	7.1	1	47
0.1	7.6	1	63
1.8	45.4	7.9	151
0.8	45.7	10.7	19
0.3	9.8	3.2	166
0.2	12.2	1.4	60
0.1	14.3	1.1	45
0.1	5.4	1.1	61
0.1	8.4	1.2	28

FOOD	PORTION	CALORIES	FAT (G)
MEATS			
Beef			
Corned beef hash, canned	1 cup	398	24.9
Ground, broiled, regular	3 oz	248	16.5
Ground, broiled, lean	3 oz	238	15
Ground, broiled, extra-lean	3 oz	225	13.4
Steak, rib eye, lean, broiled	3 oz	191	10
Steak, porterhouse, lean, broiled	3 oz	185	9.2
Steak, T-bone, lean, broiled	3 oz	182	8.8
Steak, filet mignon, lean, broiled	3 oz	179	8.5
Steak, sirloin, wedge bone, lean, broiled	3 oz	166	6.1
Liver, braised	3 oz	137	4.2
Steak, top round, lean, broiled	3 oz	153	4.2

SATURATED FAT (G)	% CALORIES FROM FAT	% CALORIES FROM SATURATED FAT	CHOLESTEROL (mg)
11.9	56.3	26.9	73
6.5	59.9	23.6	86
5.9	56.7	22.3	86
5.3	53.6	21.2	84
4	47.1	18.8	68
3.7	44.8	18	68
3.5	43.5	17.3	68
3.2	42.7	16.1	71
2.4	33.1	13	76
1.6	27.6	10.5	331
1.4	24.7	8.2	71

FOOD	PORTION	CALORIES	FAT (G)
Lamb			
Rib roast, crown, lean, roasted	3 oz	197	11.3
Pork			
Spareribs, lean, braised	3 oz	337	25.8
Bacon, smoked	3 medium slices (about ¾ oz total)	109	9.4
Ham, cured, roasted	3 oz	140	6.5
Bacon, Canadian	2 medium slices (about 1½ oz total)	86	3.9

MILK AND MILK PRODUCTS

FOOD	PORTION	CALORIES	FAT (G)
Eggnog	½ cup	171	9.5
Milk, whole	1 cup	157	8.9
Milk, whole, chocolate	1 cup	208	8.5
Sour cream, regular	2 Tbsp	62	6
Cream, light	2 Tbsp	59	5.8
Milk, 2%	1 cup	121	4.7
Cream, flavored	1 tsp	60	3
Half-and-half	2 Tbsp	39	3.5
Milk, 1%	1 cup	102	2.6

SATURATED FAT (G)	% CALORIES FROM FAT	% CALORIES FROM SATURATED FAT	CHOLESTEROL (mg)
4.1	51.6	18.7	75
10	68.9	26.7	103
3.3	77.6	27.2	16
2.2	41.8	14.1	48
1.3	40.8	13.6	27
5.7	50	30	75
5.6	51	32.1	35
5.3	36.8	22.9	31
3.8	87.1	55.2	13
3.6	88.5	54.9	20
2.9	35	21.6	18
2.5	45	37.5	0
2.2	80.8	50.8	11
1.6	22.9	14.1	10

FOOD	PORTION	CALORIES	FAT (G)
Milk, 1%, chocolate	1 cup	158	2.5
Sour cream, reduced-fat	2 Tbsp	35	2
Buttermilk	1 cup	99	2.2
Milk, fat-free	1 cup	86	0.4
Sour cream, fat-free	2 Tbsp	30	0

POULTRY

FOOD	PORTION	CALORIES	FAT (G)
Chicken breast, fried in batter, with skin	½ (about 5 oz)	364	18.5
Duck, roasted, without skin	3 oz	171	9.5
Chicken, drumstick, fried in batter, with skin	1 (about 3 oz)	193	11.3
Turkey, dark meat, roasted, with skin	3 oz	188	9.8
Turkey, light meat, roasted, with skin	3 oz	168	7.1
Chicken breast, fried in batter, without skin	½ (about 3 oz)	161	4.1
Chicken breast, roasted, without skin	½ (about 3 oz)	142	3.1

SATURATED FAT (G)	% CALORIES FROM FAT	% CALORIES FROM SATURATED FAT	CHOLESTEROL (mg)
1.5	14.2	8.5	7
1.5	51.4	38.6	10
1.3	20	11.8	9
0.3	4.2	3.1	4
0	0	0	2
4.9	45.7	12.1	119
3.6	50	18.9	76
3	52.7	14	62
3	46.9	14.4	76
2	38	10.7	65
1.1	22.9	6.1	78
0.9	19.6	5.7	73

FOOD	PORTION	CALORIES	FAT (G)
Turkey, breast, prebasted, roasted, without skin	3 oz	107	2.9
Turkey, dark meat, roasted, without skin	3 oz	32	1.2
Turkey, light meat, roasted, without skin	3 oz	34	0.7

SALAD DRESSINGS

FOOD	PORTION	CALORIES	FAT (G)
Blue cheese, regular	2 Tbsp	170	17
Caesar	2 Tbsp	170	18
Blue cheese, low-fat	2 Tbsp	80	8
French	2 Tbsp	120	12
Oil and vinegar	2 Tbsp	110	11
Honey Dijon	2 Tbsp	130	10
Italian	2 Tbsp	100	10
Ranch, regular	2 Tbsp	140	14
Thousand Island	2 Tbsp	110	10
Ranch, low-fat	2 Tbsp	80	7
Blue cheese, fat-free	2 Tbsp	35	0
Ranch, fat-free	2 Tbsp	45	0

SATURATED FAT (G)	% CALORIES FROM FAT	% CALORIES FROM SATURATED FAT	CHOLESTEROL (mg)
0.8	24.4	6.7	36
0.4	33.8	11.3	15
0.2	18.5	5.3	15
3	90	15.9	10
2.5	95.3	13.2	0
2	90	22.5	0
2	90	15	0
2	90	16.4	0
1.5	69.2	10.4	0
1.5	90	13.5	0
1.5	90	9.6	10
1.5	81.8	12.3	10
0.5	78.8	5.6	0
0	0	0	0
0	0	0	0

INDEX